Pocket Guide to Pediatric Assessment

Pocket Guide to Pediatric Assessment

Joyce Engel, R.N., M.Ed.
Assistant Professor
School of Nursing
University of Lethbridge
Lethbridge, Alberta, Canada

Second Edition

with 84 illustrations

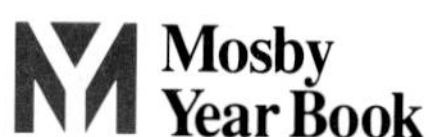

St. Louis Baltimore Boston Chicago London Philadelphia Sydney Toronto

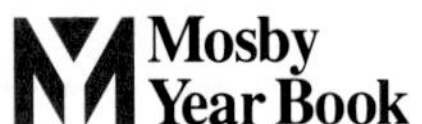

Dedicated to Publishing Excellence

Editor: Don Ladig
Managing Editor: Robin Carter
Project Manager: Gayle May Morris
Designer: Jeanne Wolfgeher
Cover Photograph: Bill Leslie Photography, Inc.

SECOND EDITION

Printed in the United States of America

Mosby–Year Book, Inc.
11830 Westline Industrial Drive, St. Louis, Missouri 63146

Library of Congress Cataloging in Publication Data

Engel, Joyce.
Pocket guide to pediatric assessment / Joyce Engel. — 2nd ed.
p. cm.
Includes bibliographical references and index.
ISBN 0-8016-6691-0
1. Children—Medical examinations—Handbooks, manuals, etc. 2. Children—Diseases—Diagnosis—Handbooks, manuals, etc. 3. Physical diagnosis—Handbooks, manuals, etc. 4. Pediatric nursing—Handbooks, manuals, etc. I. Title.
[DNLM: 1. Nursing Assessment—handbooks. 2. Pediatric Nursing—handbooks. 3. Physical Examination—in infancy & childhood—handbooks. WY 39 E57p]
RJ50.E64 1993
618.92'0075—dc20
DNLM/DLC
for Library of Congress 92-49621
CIP

93 94 95 96 97 CL/DC 9 8 7 6 5 4 3 2 1

Consultants

Barbara W. Berg, RN, PNP, MN
Head Nurse,
Rose Children's Center at Rose Medical Center,
Denver, Colorado

Heather Brookwell-Rueber, RN, MSN
Instructor,
Medicine Hat College,
Medicine Hat, Alberta
Canada

Terry Fugate, RN, BSN
Formerly Adjunct and Associate Faculty,
Texas Tech University,
Health Sciences Center,
Lubbock, Texas

Sarah G. Fuller, RN, CPNP, PhD
Associate Professor,
College of Nursing,
University of South Carolina,
Columbia, South Carolina

Sandra L. Gardner, RN, MS, PNP
Director,
Professional Outreach Consultation,
Aurora, Colorado

Marilyn B. Hartsell, RN, MSN
Coordinator,
Tri-Regional Education and Networking Development System,
University of Delaware,
Newark, Delaware

Karen Helverson, RN, MN
Director,
School of Nursing,
Medicine Hat College,
Medicine Hat, Alberta
Canada

Christina Bergh Jackson, RN, CPNP, MSN
Pediatric Nurse Practitioner,
Pennsylvania School of the Deaf,
Philadelphia, Pennsylvania;
Instructor,
Eastern College,
St. Davids, Pennsylvania

Carol A. Kilmon, RN, CPNP, MSN, PhD
Assistant Professor,
The University of Texas Medical Branch,
Galveston, Texas

Mary Ann Norton, RNC, CPNP, PhD
Associate Professor,
North Michigan University,
Marquette, Michigan

Margaret C. Slota, RN, MN
Pediatrics Consultant,
Pittsburgh, Pennsylvania

Janet F. Sullivan, RN, C, PhD
Clinical Associate Professor,
Parent Child Health Nursing,
State of New York Health Sciences Center,
Stony Brook, New York

Preface

Like the first edition, this second edition of Pocket Guide to Pediatric Assessment does not guarantee a sense of humor. It does, however, continue to recognize that the nurse, whether at a student or graduate level, requires accessible and specific information when beginning or expanding skills in the assessment of children.

Organization and Approach

The book retains its practical, systematic, and clear, direct approach to the assessment of children. Essential skills and knowledge related to assessment are presented within a developmentally based framework. The practitioner is introduced to general tips and methods in approaching and assessing children and to findings that are relevant to common health problems and practices in children. Clinical alerts delineate important deviations, thereby assisting in clinical decision making. Nursing diagnoses complete the first step in the nursing process and assist in making the leap from observation, palpation, percussion, and asculation to meaningful conclusions.

New to this Edition

This second edition of Pocket Guide to Pediatric Assessment adds to comprehensiveness in assessment through the addition of chapters on family assessment and child abuse. In keeping with the general thrust of the book, family assessment guidelines are practical and prefaced with a broad overview of theory underlying families and assessment. Sample questions are presented in each section and important findings, normal and abnormal, are presented for easy reference. The chapter on child abuse, which follows all other chapters on assessment, recognizes that abuse can be multisystem and involves developmental and psychosocial aspects of a child's functioning.

Further changes and additions to the second edition of Pocket Guide to Pediatric Assessment include a section on documentation of findings, current immunization schedules, and the most recent information related to developmental screening. Content has been added that updates findings pertinent to children with immune deficiencies and to children born to mothers who abuse drugs. Every effort has been made to include information that is critical to responsive, knowledgable assessment of children within current contexts.

• • •

The overall aim of this book continues to be the provision of accessible information that can be readily and specifically applied to the assessment of children. I appreciate the feedback from student and graduate nurses of diverse expertise, from the literature, and from my own children, who have kept me true to the practicalities and imperatives in pediatric health care and to the importance of responding to children with exquisite knowledge of their childness.

JEngel

Contents

V. Concluding the Assessment

Appendices

PART

I

HEALTH HISTORY

Beginning the Assessment

1

The focus of this text is on health assessment of the child, beginning with the 1-month-old infant and ending with the teenager in late adolescence. Although the physical assessment process is broken down into evaluations of the various body systems, the nurse need not adopt a fragmented approach to physical assessment. In fact, physical assessment is continuous and occurs during the health interview, when the nurse is also able to observe the infant or child.

Assessment is facilitated for child, parent (if present), and examiner if a rapport is established early. It may not be possible to erase all of a child's apprehension or discomfort, but setting up a relationship of trust and communication can help make the assessment a more positive experience.

Guidelines for Communicating with Children

- Ask the parents how the child usually copes with new or stressful situations. Knowing how the child might react enables the nurse to plan specific interventions to facilitate communication.
- Ask the parents what they have told the child about the health care encounter. The preparation children receive, especially males, is often inadequate or inappropriate. If so, more time may be needed to prepare the child before beginning any aspect of the health assessment requiring active participation.
- Observe the child's behavior for clues to readiness. A child who is ready to participate in assessment will ask questions, make eye contact, describe past experiences, touch equipment, or detach willingly from the parent.
- Consider the child's developmental level and attention span and use an imaginative approach when planning the examination.

- If a child is having difficulty accepting the assessment
    - Talk to the parent, ignoring the child
    - Compliment the child
    - Play a game (such as peek-a-boo) or tell a story
    - Use the third-person linguistic form: "Sometimes a guy can get really scared when his blood pressure is taken."
    - Briefly perform the technique on the parent first.
- Encourage the child to ask questions during assessment, but do not pressure to do so. This allows the child some control over the situation.
- Explain the assessment process in terms consistent with the child's developmental level.
- Use concrete terms rather than technical information, particularly with younger children: "I can hear you breathing in and out," not "I am auscultating your chest."
- Present small amounts of information at a time. A rule of thumb is that no more than three items should be presented at once.
- Make expectations known clearly and simply: "I want you to be very still."
- *Do not offer choice where there is none.*
- Offer honest praise: "I know that hurt. You held your tummy very still." A positive experience helps to build coping skills and self-esteem.

Communicating with Infants

Infants (1 to 18 months) primarily communicate through nonverbal vocalization and crying and respond to nonverbal communication behaviors of adults, such as holding, rocking, and patting. It is useful to observe the parent's or significant other's interpretation of the infant's nonverbal cues and the nonverbal communications of the parents. These established communication patterns can aid the nurse in setting up rapport with the infant.

Young infants respond well to gentle physical contact with any adult, but older infants are frequently wary of adults other than their parents. If it is necessary to handle the older infant, do so firmly and without preparatory gestures such as holding out hands or coaxing the child to come. As much as possible, carry out the assessment in a way that allows the infant to either keep the parent in view or to be held by the parent. Infants should be allowed security objects such as blankets and pacifiers, if they have them.

Communicating with Toddlers

Toddlers (18 months to 3 years) have not yet acquired the ability to effectively communicate verbally. Their communication is rich with expressive nonverbal gestures and simple verbal communications. Pushing the examiner's hand away and crying can be an eloquent expression of fear, anxiety, or lack of knowledge. Toddlers accept the verbal communications of others literally, so that saying, "I can see all the way to your tummy button when you open your mouth" will mean just that to toddlers. Toddlers have the beginnings of memory and make believe but they are unable to understand abstractions and become frustrated and frightened by phrases that seem ordinary to adults.

Communication with toddlers requires that the nurse use short, concrete terms. Explanations and descriptions need to be repeated several times. Visual aids such as puppets and dolls assist explanations. Children of this age attribute magical qualities to inanimate objects, so it is useful to allow them to handle instruments and to tell them exactly, in concrete terms, what the instrument does and how it feels. The use of comfort objects should be encouraged throughout the assessment.

Communicating with Preschool-Aged Children

Although preschoolers (3 to 6 years) generally use more sophisticated verbal communications, their reasoning is intuitive. Therefore many of the guidelines for communicating with toddlers apply to preschoolers as well. Because of the preschooler's increased verbal communication abilities, the nurse can successfully indicate to the child how and when cooperation is desired. The older preschooler, in particular, likes to conform and may be interested in the purpose of various parts of the assessment. Allowing the preschooler to handle the equipment eases fears and helps to answer questions about how the equipment is used.

Preschool-aged children are often very modest and should be exposed minimally during examination. They need to know exactly what is being examined and benefit from opportunities for questions.

Communicating with School-Aged Children

School-aged children (6 to 12 years) think in concrete terms but at a more sophisticated level. Generally they have had enough contact with health care personnel that they can rely on past experiences to guide them. Depending on the quality of their past experiences, they may appear shy or reticent during health assessment. Frequently they may fear injury or embarrassment. Allowing time for composure and privacy (perhaps even from parents) aids in communication. Reassurance and third-person speech are helpful in eliciting fears and anxieties and in allowing the child to express hurt.

The purpose of the health assessment should be related to the child's condition. It is useful to determine what the child already knows about the health contact and to proceed from there. Simple medical diagrams and teaching dolls are useful in explaining the assessment process. Specific information should be given about body parts affected by the assessment.

Children of this age are often curious about the function of equipment and its usefulness. An appropriate response to "How can you tell what my temperature is from the thermometer?" might be "Your body heat pushes the silver up the glass tube. I can read how far the silver has been pushed up the scale on the tube."

Communicating with Adolescents

Adolescents (12 years and older) use sophisticated verbal communication, although their behavior may not necessarily indicate an advanced level of communication, cognition, or maturity. Adolescents may respond to verbal approaches with monosyllables, reticence, anger, or other behaviors. The nurse must avoid the tendency to respond to less than desirable social behaviors with prying, confrontation, or judgmental attitudes. Easing into the initial contact with discussion of irrelevant topics can give the apprehensive adolescent time for self-composure.

It is helpful to ask the adolescent what he or she knows about the health contact and to explain the rationale for the health assessment. Adolescents may be concerned about privacy and confidentiality, and opportunity should be provided for completing some or all of the assessment without the presence of the parent.

Adolescents tend to be preoccupied with body image and function, and when appropriate should be given feedback from the assessment. Diagrams and models can enhance feedback. Although adolescents have a high level of comprehension and vocabulary, they may not consistently function at higher levels of cognition, and the nurse must avoid the tendency to become too abstract, too detailed, and too technical. The self-conscious adolescent may be reluctant to ask for clarification of an explanation that has not been understood.

Communicating with Parents

Parents are often an integral part of the health assessment of an infant or child. Parents are the primary source of information about the young child. The information that parents give can be considered reliable in most instances, because of close contact with their children.

Broad questions are useful, especially in eliciting responses in sensitive areas, because the parent can assume control over the direction of the response: "Tell me what Jason did at 2 years" is less threatening than "Did Jason talk when he was 2?" or "Did you have trouble disciplining Jason when he was 2?" More focused and closed questions should be saved for later in the assessment process when specific information is desired.

The use of silence and of listening is essential in reassuring parents that what they are about to say is worthwhile. In a supportive, attentive atmosphere parents often communicate information and feelings that may have little to do with the current problem but have great significance in the overall care of the child.

The parents are members of the health team. If they believe the child has a problem, their concern must be treated seriously. The parents and the nurse must agree that the problem exists. Once agreement exists, the nurse can ask how the parents have tried to solve the problem. This approach reinforces the worth of the parents' solutions. Having accomplished this, the nurse can help the parents to find alternative solutions for the problem. Occasionally parents will select alternatives that are not preferred. If the alternative will not harm the child, it is best to allow the parents to carry out their plan.

The nurse must avoid the temptation to inundate the parents with anticipatory guidance. Parents need recognition, praise, and reassurance for their strengths. Too much information and advice can intimidate parents and effectively shut down communication.

Establishing Setting for Health History

The health interview provides an ideal opportunity for the establishment of communication and rapport and usually is the first step in an assessment. The interview should be conducted in a room that is private, bright, and nonthreatening. Toys and drawing materials are useful for distracting the young child, so that the parent can give the interviewer fuller attention.

Before beginning the health interview, nurses must introduce themselves and ask the names of family members. Family members are then addressed by name. Unless an infant, the child is usually included in the interview; the extent of involvement varies with age.

Nurses must clarify their roles in the assessment process because in some health settings many health practitioners see the child. The purposes of the health interview and physical assessment are clarified, because parents may wonder about the relevance of the information they are about to give. Parents, and the child, as appropriate, are also told who has access to the information and are assured as to the limits of access. Once the parameters of the interview and physical assessment have been set, the parents are better able to decide how and what they wish to communicate.

Dimensions of a History

2

Obtaining a health history is an important component of the health assessment process. The health interview assists in establishing rapport with the parent and child, provides data from which tentative diagnoses can be made, and offers an opportunity for the nurse and family to establish goals.

The purposes and extent of the health interview varies with the nature of the health care contact. For example, in an emergency situation it is necessary to focus on the chief complaint and the details of past health care contacts. The prenatal and postnatal histories and the psychosocial dimensions can be left for later. When a child has repeated contacts with a health care facility, it is necessary only to update a health history if it has been completed on initial contact. The course of an interview must be modified to fit the situation and the setting.

Guidelines for Interviewing Parents and Children

- Follow principles of communication (see Chapter 1) during the interview.
- Before beginning the interview the nurse must thoroughly understand the purposes of the health history and of the questions that are asked.
- If a specific illness is the reason for the interview, knowledge of the diagnosis helps to focus questions related to the chief complaint. The nurse must also be alert to concerns raised by the parent or child that are not related to the diagnosis.
- Explain the purpose of the interview, before starting, to the parents and to the child. Cooperation and sharing are more likely if the parents understand that the questions ensure better care for their child.

- Write brief notations about specific details. *Do not try to write finished sentences,* and *keep writing to a minimum.* The flow of contact is lost if the nurse spends an extended amount of time writing or in staring at a form.
- Know what information is necessary so that the parents and child are not asked for the same type of information repeatedly. *Repeat questions only if further clarification is desired.*
- Give broad openings at the beginning of the interview, such as "Tell me why you came to see me today?" Use direct questions, such as "Are the stools watery?" to assist the parent to focus on specific details.
- Do not interrupt the parent or child.
- Accept what is being said. Nodding, reestablishing eye contact, or saying uh-huh provides encouragement to continue.
- Listen, and attend to nonverbal cues. The presenting complaint may have little to do with the real concern.
- Convey empathy and an unhurried attitude. Sit, at eye level, if possible.
- Ensure mutual understanding. *Clarify* if unsure, and summarize for the parent and child what has been understood.
- Integrate the child when possible. Even the very young can answer the question "What do you like to eat?"
- Be sensitive to the need to separately interview parents and child, particularly if the child is an adolescent.

Information for Comprehensive History

Information	Comment
Date of History Identifying Data	
Include name, nickname, parents' names, home telephone number, number where parents can be reached during working hours, child's date of birth, age (months, years), sex, race, language spoken, language understood.	Much of this information may already be on a child's nameplate or chart.

Information	Comment
Source of Referral, if Any	
Source of Information	
Include judgment as to reliability of information.	
Chief Complaint	
Use broad opening statements, such as "What concerns bring you here today?" Record parents' or child's own words: "Diarrhea since Saturday."	Note who has identified the chief complaint. In some instances a schoolteacher or physician may have expressed the concern. Agreement between parents and another referral source is important to care.
Present Illness	
Include a chronologic narrative of the chief complaint. The narrative answers questions related to *where* (location), *what* (quality, factors that aggravate or relieve symptoms), *when* (onset, duration, frequency), and *how much* (intensity, severity). The parent or child should also be asked about associated manifestations. Include significant negatives: "The parent denies that the child has experienced undue fatigue, bruising, or joint tenderness." Use direct questions to focus on specific details, as necessary.	Parents may need assistance in sorting out details. Prior knowledge of diagnosis aids in planning specific questions. **Clinical Alert** Persistent denial in the face of unexplained or vaguely defined injuries may signal child abuse.
Past Medical History	
General state of health	
Inquire about appetite, recent weight losses or gains, fatigue, stresses.	Do not include information that may have been elicited for chief complaint or present illness.

Information	Comment
Birth history	
Include prenatal history (maternal health, infections, medications taken, abnormal bleeding, weight gain, duration of pregnancy, attitudes toward pregnancy, birth, duration of labor, type of delivery, complications, birth weight, condition of infant at birth), and neonatal history (respiratory distress, cyanosis, jaundice, seizures, poor feeding, patterns of sleeping).	Birth history is especially important if the child is younger than 2 years or is experiencing developmental or neurologic problems.
Feeding	
For infants, include type of feeding (bottle, breast, solid foods), frequency of feedings, quantity of feeds, responses to feeding, and specific problems with feeding (colic, regurgitation, lethargy). For children, include self-feeding abilities, likes and dislikes, appetite, and amounts of food taken.	Guidelines for a more complete nutritional history are supplied in Chapter 4.
Previous illnesses, operations, or injuries	
Include dates of hospitalizations, reasons for hospitalizations, and responses to illnesses.	Knowing how a child has reacted in past hospitalizations can help in planning interventions for a current hospitalization.

Information	Comment
Childhood illnesses	
Include the common communicable diseases, such as measles, mumps, and chickenpox. Inquire about recent contacts with persons with communicable diseases.	
Immunizations	
Include specific details about immunizations (dates, types) and untoward reactions. If a child has not been immunized, note the reason. Note desensitization procedures, e.g., measles/mumps/rubella (MMR).	MMR vaccine contains chick embryo tissue that may trigger a reaction in egg-sensitive patients.
Current medications	
Include prescription and nonprescription drugs, dose, frequency, and time of last dose.	
Allergies	
Include agent *and* reaction.	Knowing the reaction is useful since reactions may not be indicative of allergic manifestations.
Growth and Development	
Physical	
Include approximate height and weight at 1, 2, 5, and 10 years, and tooth eruption/loss.	A thorough history of growth and development is important in planning nursing interventions appropriate to the child's level and in screening for developmental and neurologic problems. A social history can identify the need for anticipatory guidance.
Developmental history	
Include ages at which child rolled over, sat alone, crawled, walked, spoke first words, spoke first sentences, and dressed without help.	

Information	Comment
Social history	
Include toileting (age at which daytime and nighttime control were achieved or current level of control, enuresis, enioparesis, self-toileting abilities, terminology used); sleep (amount and patterns during day and night, bedtime rituals and security objects, fears, and nightmares); speech (lisping, stuttering, intelligibility); sexuality (relationships with members of opposite sex, inquisitiveness about sexual information and activity, type of information given child); schooling (grade level in school, academic achievement, adjustment to school); habits (thumb sucking, nail biting, pica, head banging); discipline (methods used, child's response to discipline); and personality and temperament (congeniality, aggressiveness, temper tantrums, withdrawal, relationships with peers and family). Children and adolescents should be asked if they ever feel sad or "down." If yes, they should be asked if they have ever thought of killing themselves.	Behavior and temperament may provide important diagnostic and intervention information. Children with hearing impairments as well as school-aged children who experience recurrent abdominal pain are more likely to have difficult temperaments. Children with chronic cardiac disease are more intense, withdrawn, and more negative in mood than healthy children. Boys from violent home environments tend to bully, be argumentative, and have temper tantrums and short attention spans. Girls from violent homes tend to be anxious or depressed, to cling, and to be perfectionists. Infants born to mothers on cocaine exhibit sleep problems.

A

Male

Female

Died

A&W Alive and well

Adopted

Divorced or separated

Living together

Abortion or miscarriage

Stillborn male

Miscarriage, sex unknown

Patient

B

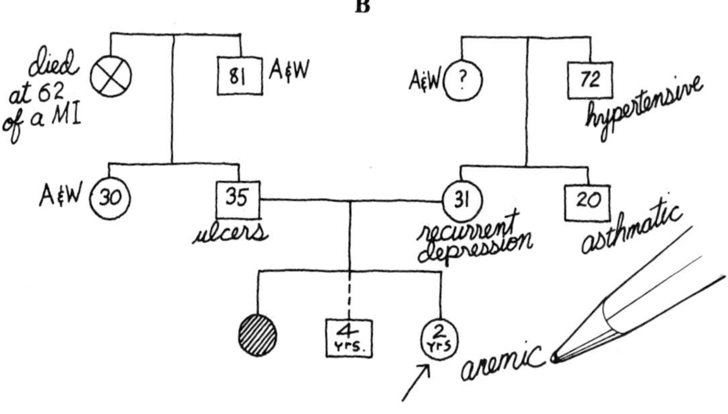

Figure 2-1
Constructing a genogram. **A,** Symbols used in a genogram. **B,** Sample genogram.

Information	Comment
Family History	
Include the ages and health of immediate family members, familial diseases, presence and types of congenital anomalies, consanguinity of parents, occupations and education of parents, and family interactions. Inquire about living conditions (type of family dwelling and neighborhood).	A genogram (Figure 2-1) is useful for showing the relationships, ages, and health of family members. See Chapter 3 for a more detailed family assessment. Needs of health care programs should be balanced with needs of families. Parents identify their main needs as information about diagnosis, effect of diagnosis on development, information about treatment, and effect of condition on sexuality of child.
Systems Review	
1. General 2. Integument 3. Head and neck 4. Ears 5. Eyes 6. Face and nose 7. Thorax and lungs 8. Cardiovascular 9. Abdominal 10. Genitourinary/reproductive 11. Musculoskeletal 12. Neurologic	Questions appropriate for each system are included under the heading of "Preparation" in chapters of the textbook.

Family Assessment

3

Assessment of the family includes exploration of structure, function, and developmental stage. While family *therapy* is within the practice realm of those with special education and supervision, assessment is appropriate for practitioners with general preparation.

The assessment guidelines outlined in this chapter are adapted from those outlined by Wright and Leahey (1984) in the Calgary Family Assessment Model (CFAM) and reflect its strongly supported systems approach to family care.

Rationale

The family should be viewed as interacting, complex elements. The decisions and activities of one family member affect the others and the family has an impact on the individual. Understanding family members' interactions and communications, family norms and expectations, how decisions are made, and how the family balances individual and family needs enables the nurse to understand the family's responses and needs during times of stress and well-being. This understanding can enrich the relationship between the nurse and family. The nurse's positive, proactive responses to family concerns and capabilities can serve to help the family promote the development and well-being of its members.

General Concepts Related to Assessment

The primary premise in family systems assessment is that individuals are best understood in the context of their families. Studying a child and a parent as separate units does not constitute family assessment because it neglects observation of interaction. The parents and children are part of subsystems within a larger family system, which in turn is part of a larger subsystem. Changes in any one of these system components affect the other components, a characteristic that has been likened to the impact of wind or motion upon the pieces of a mobile.

The analogy of a mobile is useful for considering a second concept in family systems assessment. When piece A of the mobile strikes piece B, piece B may rebound and strike piece A with increased energy. Piece A affects piece B and piece B affects A. Circular causality assumes that behavior is reciprocal; each family member's behavior influences the others. If mother responds angrily to her toddler because he turned on the hot water tap while her infant was in the tub, the toddler reciprocates with a response that further influences the mother. It is important to remain open to the multiple interpretations of reality within a family, recognizing that family members may not fully realize how their behavior affects others or how others affect them.

All systems have boundaries. Knowledge of the family's boundaries may enable the nurse to predict the level of social support that the family may perceive and receive. Families with rigid, closed boundaries may have few contacts with the community suprasystem and may require tremendous assistance to network appropriately for help. Conversely, families with very loose, permeable boundaries may be caught between many opinions as they seek to make care decisions. Members within family systems may similarly experience extremely closed or permeable boundaries. In enmeshed families, boundaries between parent and child subsystems may be blurred to the extent that children adopt inappropriate parental roles. In more rigid families, the boundaries between adult and child subsystems may be so closed that the developing child is unable to assume more mature roles.

Families attempt to maintain balances between change and stability. The crisis of illness temporarily may produce a state of great change within a family. Efforts at stability such as emphatic attempts at maintenance of usual feeding routines during the illness of an infant may seem paradoxical to the period of change. However, both change and stability can and do coexist in family systems. Overwhelming change or rigid equilibrium, however, can contribute to and be symptomatic of severe family dysfunction. Sustained change usually produces a new level of balance as the family regroups and reorganizes to cope with the change.

Stages in Family Development

Change and stability are integral concepts in development. Like individuals, families experience a developmental sequence, which can be divided into eight distinct stages.

Stage One: Marriage (Joining of Families)

Marriage entails the combining of families of origin as well as of individuals. Essential to the successful resolution of this stage is the establishment of couple identity and the negotiation of new relationships with the families of origin.

Stage Two: Families with Infants

This stage begins with the birth of the first child and involves integration of the infant into the family, design and acceptance of new roles, and maintenance of the spousal relationship. A decrease in marital satisfaction is common during this stage, especially if the infant is ill or has a handicapping condition.

Stage Three: Families with Preschoolers

Stage three begins when the eldest child is 3 years of age and involves socialization of the child(ren) and successful adjustment to separation by parents and child(ren).

Stage Four: Families with School-aged Children

This stage begins when the eldest child begins elementary or primary school (at about 6 years). While all stages are perceived by some families as especially stressful, others report this as a particularly stressful stage. Tasks involve establishment of peer relationships by the children and adjustment to peer and other external influences by the parents.

Stage Five: Families with Teenagers

This stage begins when the eldest child is 13 years of age and is viewed by some as an intense period of turmoil. Stage five focuses on the increasing autonomy and individualization of the child, a return to midlife and career issues for parents, and increasing recognition by parents of their predicament as the sandwich generation.

Stage Six: Families as Launching Centers

Stage six begins when the first child leaves home and continues until the youngest child departs. During this time, the couple realigns the marital relationship while they and the child(ren) adjust to new roles as parents and separate adults.

Stage Seven: Middle-Aged Families

Stage seven begins when the last child leaves home and continues until a parent retires. Successful resolution depends on development of independent interests within a newly reconstituted couple identity, inclusion of new and extended family relationships, and coming to terms with disabilities and deaths in the older generation.

Stage Eight: Aging Families

This stage begins with retirement and ends with the death of the spouses. It is marked by concern with development of retirement roles, maintenance of individual/couple relationships with aging, and preparation for death.

Guidelines for Communicating with Families

- Display a sincere sense of warmth, caring, and encouragement.
- Demonstrate neutrality; perceptions of partiality toward particular family members may interfere with assessment and assistance.
- Use active and reflective listening.
- Convey a sense of cooperation and partnership with the family. Promote participatory decision making.
- Promote the competencies of the family.
- Encourage the family's use of natural support networks.

Assessment of the Family

Assessment of the family usually involves the entire family except when the infant or child is too ill to participate.

Assessment	Findings
Internal Structure	
Use a genogram (see Chapter 2) to diagram family structure. The genogram is often useful in helping the family to clarify information related to family composition.	
Family composition Refers to everyone in the household. Ask who is in the family.	**Clinical Alert** Losses or additions to families may result in crisis.
Rank order Refers to the arrangement of children according to age and gender.	Family position is thought to influence relationships and even careers. Eldest children are considered more conscientious, perfectionistic; middle children are sometimes considered nonconformist, and to have many friends; and youngest children are sometimes seen as precocious, less responsible with resources, and playful. **Clinical Alert** Frequent references to rank order ("She's the eldest") may signify a role assignment that is uncomfortable for the individual who is involved.
Subsystems Smaller units in the family marked by sex, role, interests, or age. Ask if the family has special smaller groups.	**Clinical Alert** A child who acts as a parent surrogate may signify family dysfunction or abuse.

Assessment	Findings
Boundaries Refers to who is part of what system or subsystem. Need to consider if family boundaries and subsystems are closed, open, rigid, or permeable. Ask who the family members approach with concerns.	**Clinical Alert** A family with rigid boundaries may become distanced or disengaged from others. Disengagement may also occur within families; these families are characterized by little intrafamilial communication and highly autonomous members.
External Structure Can be visually represented with an ecomap (see Figure 3-1). Culture Way of life for a group. Ask if other languages are spoken. Ask how long family has lived in area/country. Ask if family identifies with a particular ethnic group. Ask how ethnic background influences their lifestyle. May impact significantly on care.	The internal and external structures of a family, as well as parenting practices, are affected by ethnicity. For example, Native American Indians discipline through observational learning rather than through coercive control.

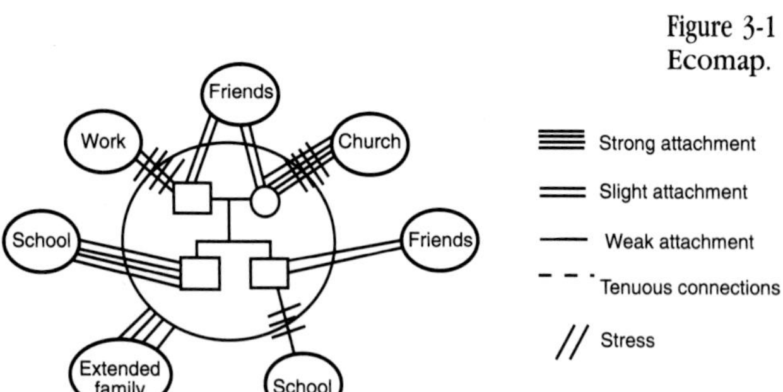

Figure 3-1 Ecomap.

Assessment	Findings
Religion	
Influences family values and beliefs.	For example, in families who are Jehovah's Witnesses, blood transfusions are opposed. Christian Scientists believe that healing is a religious function and oppose drugs, blood transfusions, and extensive physical examinations.
May impact on care of the child/infant.	
Ask if family is involved in a church or if they identify with a particular religious group.	
How religion is a part of their life.	
Observe for religious icons and artifacts in the home.	
Social class status and mobility	
Mold family values.	
Inquire about work moves, satisfaction, and aspirations.	
Environment	**Clinical Alert**
Refers to home, neighborhood, and community.	Chipped paint, heavy street traffic, uncertain water supplies, and sanitation can all affect family health.
Refers to adequacy and safety of home, school, recreation, and transportation.	
May impact on family's abilities to visit and ongoing care.	
Extended family	
Refers to families of origin and step-relatives.	Extended family may need to be involved in care if contact is significant.
Ask about contacts (who? frequency? significance?) with extended family members.	

Assessment	Findings
Family development Use age and school placement of oldest child to delineate stage. Questions evolve from the developmental stage of the family. For Stage two, the practitioner might inquire as to the differences noticed since the birth of an infant.	**Clinical Alert** A family that resists change may become stuck in a stage. The adolescent, for example, may be treated as a young child, producing great distress. Family breakdown and divorce affect the family differently depending on the timing in the family cycle.
Instrumental functioning Refers to the routine mechanics of eating, dressing, sleeping. Inquire about concerns with accomplishment of daily tasks.	**Clinical Alert** An ill or disabled child may significantly alter the family's pattern of activities and abilities to carry out activities.
Expressive functioning Refers to the affective issues and is useful in delineating functional families and those families who are experiencing distress and who would benefit from intervention or referral.	**Clinical Alert** A family may refuse to show emotion appropriately or allow members to do so, which can suggest dysfunction. In alcoholic families, for example, members may show an unusually bland response to extremes in circumstances or behavior.
Emotional communication Range and type of emotions expressed in a family. Inquire how intense emotions such as anger and sadness are expressed and who is most expressive. Ask who provides comfort in the family. When something new is to be tried, who provides support?	**Clinical Alert** Expression may be narrow, rigid, and inappropriate in dysfunctional families.

Assessment	Findings
Verbal communication Verbal communication addresses the clarity, directness, openness and direction of communication. Can be observed during the interview. Indirect communication may be clarified by asking questions such as "What is your mom telling you?" Observe congruence of verbal and nonverbal communications. Observe if family members wait to speak until others are through. Do parents or older siblings talk down to younger children?	**Clinical Alert** Alcoholic and/or abusive families are frequently characterized by secrecy among family members and in relation to those outside the family. Triangulation refers to an indirect communication pattern in which one member communicates with another through a third member.
Circular communications Reciprocal communications that are adaptive or maladaptive. Useful in understanding communications in dyads. If a mother complains that her adolescent never listens to her, you might inquire: "So Susan ignores your instruction. What do you do then?"	
Problem solving Refers to ability of family to solve own problems. Ask who first notices problems, how decisions are made, who makes decisions.	**Clinical Alert** Dysfunctional families may tend to employ a narrow range of strategies or to consistently apply inappropriate strategies.

Assessment	Findings
Roles Focuses on established behavior patterns. Consider flexibility or rigidity of roles and whether certain idiosyncratic roles are applied to family members. ("She's always been a problem"; "He's a good kid").	**Clinical Alert** Dysfunctional families may assign narrowly prescriptive roles.
Control Refers to ways of influencing the behavior of others. May be psychological (use of communication and feelings), corporal (hugging or spanking), or instrumental (use of reinforcers such as privileges or objects). Inquire about family rules and what occurs when rules are broken. Ask who enforces family rules. Do children have a say in rules?	**Clinical Alert** Excessive control and chaos in relation to rules and cosistency of control may signify an abusive family.
Alliances/coalitions Refers to balance and intensity of relationships between or among family members.	**Clinical Alert** In sexually abusive families, the father and daughter coalition may supplant the spousal relationship.

Related Nursing Diagnoses

Anxiety: Related to situational crisis; family chaos.

Communication, impaired verbal: Related to family processes; family roles; inadequate progression of family life cycle.

Family processes, deterations in: Related to skill or knowledge deficit; situational crisis; adjustment to chronic disease; social isolation; alterations in roles.

Coping, ineffective family: Related to situational crisis; ineffective expressive functioning; social isolation.

Parenting, alterations in: Related to skill deficit; stress; inadequate progression of family life cycle.

Physical Assessment

4

The physical assessment skills are inspection, palpation, percussion, and auscultation. (The sequence in abdominal assessment is inspection, auscultation, percussion, palpation.) The acquisition of these skills requires patience, practice, and continual refinement. More detail on these skills may be found in a textbook of adult assessment skills.

Guidelines for Inspection

- Inspection is a simple but highly skilled technique.
- Inspection involves the use of sight, hearing, and smell in a systematic assessment of infants and children.
- Inspection is essential at the beginning of the health assessment to detect obvious health concerns and to establish priorities.
- Inspection should be thorough and should involve each area of the body.
- Body parts are assessed for shape, color, symmetry, odor (Table 4-1), and abnormalities.
- Careful inspection requires good lighting.

Guidelines for Palpation

- Palpation involves the use of fingers and palms to determine temperature, hydration, texture, shape, movement, and areas of tenderness.
- Warm hands before beginning palpation.
- Keep fingernails short.
- Palpate areas of tenderness last.
- Palpate with fingertips for pulsation, size, shape, texture, and hydration.

Table 4-1 Significance of common body odors

Odor	Significance
Acetone or fruity odor	May indicate diabetic acidosis
Ammonia	May indicate urinary tract infection
Fecal odor (breath or diaper area)	Associated with soiled diapers, fecal incontinence, bowel obstruction
Foul-smelling stool	May be indicative of gastroenteritis, cystic fibrosis, malabsorption syndromes
Halitosis	Associated with poor oral hygiene, dental caries or abscess, throat infection, sinusitus, constipation
Musty odor	Associated with infection underneath a cast or dressing
Sweet, thick odor	May be indicative of *Pseudomonas* infection

- Palpate with palms for vibration.
- Palpate with back of hand for temperature.
- Use conversation or games to relax child during palpation. Muscle guarding related to tension can obscure findings. Observe reactions to palpation rather than asking "Does it hurt?"
- The nurse can assist the ticklish child by first placing the child's hands on the skin and gradually sliding hands over those of the child or by having the child keep his or her hands over the nurse's during examination.

Guidelines for Percussion

- Percussion involves the use of tapping to produce sound waves, which are characterized as to intensity, pitch, duration, and quality (Table 4-2).
- Percussion may be *direct* or *indirect*.
  - *Direct* percussion involves striking the body part directly with one or two fingers.
  - *Indirect* percussion involves a pleximeter and a plexor.
    - Place the middle finger (pleximeter) of the *nondominant hand* gently against child's skin.
    - Strike the distal joint of the pleximeter with the tip of the

Table 4-2 Percussion sounds

Percussion Sound	Intensity	Pitch	Duration	Quality	Body Region Where Sound May Be Heard
Tympany	Loud	High	Moderate	Drumlike	Gastric bubble; air-filled intestine (simulate by tapping puffed out cheeks)
Resonance	Moderate to loud	Low	Long	Hollow	Lungs
Hyperresonance	Very loud	Very low	Long	Booming	Lungs with trapped air; lungs of a young child
Dullness	Soft to moderate	High	Moderate	Thudlike	Liver; fluid-filled space, such as stomach
Flatness	Soft	High	Short	Flat	Muscle

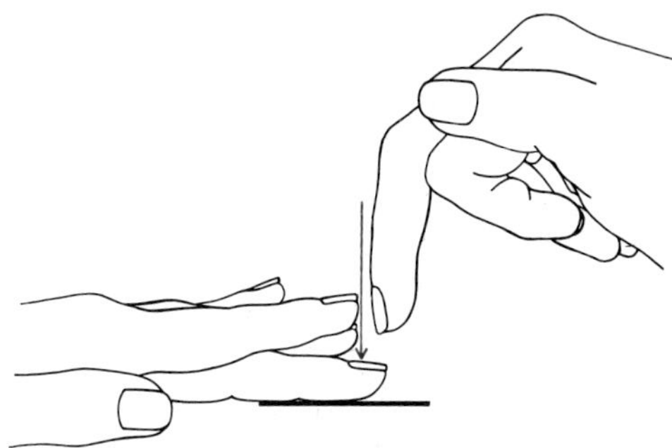

Figure 4-1
Percussion. Note position of fingers.

middle finger (plexor) of the *dominant* hand (Figure 4-1).

The blow to the pleximeter should be crisp, and the plexor must be perpendicular.

The wrist movement is essential to percussion, and must be a snapping motion.

The nail of the plexor should be short.

- Percuss from resonance to dullness.

Guidelines for Auscultation

- Auscultation is the process of listening for body sounds.
- The bell (cupped portion) of the stethoscope is used for low-pitched sounds (for example, cardiovascular sounds), and the diaphragm (flat portion) for higher pitched sounds (for example, those found in the lung and bowel).
- The stethoscope is placed firmly against the wall of the body part. The examiner must avoid pressing too firmly, causing the skin to flatten and vibrations to decrease.
- The examiner should practice in identifying normal sounds before trying to identify abnormal ones.

Preparation for Examination 5

Preparation of Environment

- Try to perform assessments somewhere other than in the child's "safe areas," when possible. "Safe areas" include the child's bedside or play area.
- Place toys, bright posters, and motifs in the examination room or area to make it look less threatening.
- Set air conditioner on low, because noisy fans can interfere with auscultation.
- Eliminate drafts from the examining area. Cold is uncomfortable for the infant or child who is minimally dressed and can alter findings. A child who is cold may appear mottled, which can also signify cardiac or respiratory disease.

Preparation of Equipment

- Ensure that all equipment is readily available.
- Place threatening or strange equipment out of easy view before beginning examination of the young child.
- Warm hands and equipment before starting examination. Equipment can be warmed with hands or with warm water.

Equipment for Physical Assessment

Cotton-tipped applicators
Paper towels and tissue
Disposable pads
Drapes
Gown for child
Gloves
Lubricant

Scale for height and weight
Tape measure
Stethoscope
Pediatric blood pressure cuff
Sphygmomanometer
Thermometers (rectal and oral)
Tongue depressor
Flashlight
Otoscope
Ophthalmoscope
Eye chart
Percussion hammer
Safety pins
Wristwatch with second hand
Physical assessment forms
Denver Developmental Screening Test (DDST) and Kit

Guidelines for Physical Assessment of Infant or Child

- Perform a general head-to-toe assessment while collecting the health history and the vital signs. General assessment assists in the establishment of priorities. Note obvious areas of distress. For example, if a child is experiencing pronounced respiratory problems, assessment of this area is a priority.
- Physical assessment is an essential component of nursing care. Children often cannot tell the caregiver what is wrong. The caregiver must be able to assess and to communicate concerns of the child arising from the assessment.
- Some aspects of a complete physical examination may be omitted during the daily assessment, depending on the child's age, health status, and the reason for the health care contact. Examples of assessments that need not always be included are height, head circumference, weight, deep tendon reflexes, and neurologic tests.
- An orderly, systematic, head-to-toe approach to examination may not be possible; it is often necessary to vary the sequence to fit the child. *Flexibility is essential;* however, all necessary aspects of an examination must eventually be covered.
- Often several observations can be made at once, because of the size of the area being examined. For example, while checking

respiratory rate it is possible to observe the type and quality of respirations, the presence or absence of retractions, the color of the trunk, and whether there is a heave under the nipple.

- Perform the least distressing aspects of the examination first. What is distressing for one age group may not be for another age group.
- Use a kind, firm approach. Tell the child what to do rather than asking for cooperation. Demonstration assists with compliance.
- Allow children to handle the equipment.
- Use both hands when possible. One hand or probing fingers may be construed as intrusive.
- Do not leave infants and children unattended on an examining room table.

Age-Related Approaches to Physical Assessment

Infant (1 to 18 Months)

- Approach the infant quietly, gently.
- Remove all clothes, except for the diaper of a male child.
- Allow the infant to be held by the parent for as much of the examination as possible.
- Distract the infant with bright toys, peek-a-boo games, and talking.
- Vary the sequence of the assessment with the infant's activity level. If the infant is quiet, obtain the pulse and respiratory rates and auscultate the lungs, heart, and abdomen at the beginning of the examination.
- Obtain the rectal temperature and perform other instrusive examinations (throat, ear) at the end of the examination.
- The parent can assist, if willing, with assessment of the ears and mouth.

Toddler (18 Months to 3 Years)

- Approach the toddler gradually. Keep physical contact to a minimum until the toddler is acquainted with you.
- Allow the toddler to remain near the parent or to be held by the parent, whenever possible.
- Introduce and use equipment gradually.
- Allow the child to handle the equipment.
- Use play to approach the child. If the child remains upset and apprehensive, carry out the assessment as quickly as possible.

- Expose the child minimally. Appropriate clothing should be removed immediately before specific assessments, and preferably by the parent.
- Sequencing of the assessment is similar to that recommended for the infant. Assessments involving the supine position may be saved until last, because children sometimes feel more vulnerable lying down.
- Encourage use of comfort objects such as blankets and stuffed toys.
- Tell the child when the assessment is completed.
- Praise the child for cooperation.

Preschool-Aged Child (3 to 6 Years)

- Allow the child to remain close to the parent.
- Allow the child to handle the equipment. Demonstrations of equipment are useful: "You can hear your own heartbeat."
- Expose the child minimally. Allow the child to take off own clothes. *This age group is particularly modest.*
- Use games to gain cooperation: "Let's see how far you can stick out your tongue."

School-Aged Child (6 to 12 Years)

- Give the older child the choice as to whether the parent is present during assessment.
- Allow the child to remove own clothing.
- Give the child a gown.
- Explain purposes of equipment: "The stethoscope is used to listen to your heartbeat."

Adolescent (12 Years and Older)

- Give the adolescent the choice as to whether the parent is present.
- Allow the adolescent to undress in private.
- Give time for the adolescent to regain self-composure before beginning the examination.
- Explain the purposes of the equipment and of assessments.
- Emphasize normalcy of development.
- Give feedback about assessment findings, if appropriate. If in doubt as to whether the sharing of particular information is appropriate, check with a more experienced caregiver.

6 Dimensions of Nutritional Assessment

Rationale

Nutritional assessment is an important initial step in nursing care and in preventive health care. It aids in identifying eating practices, misconceptions, and symptoms that can lead to nutritional problems. Because the nurse frequently has continued contact with the parents and child, the nurse often can influence dietary practices.

Establishing Weight

Weight measurement is plotted on a growth chart (see Appendix B). Normally weight remains within the same percentile from measurement to measurement. Sudden increases or decreases should be noted. Average weight and height increases for each age group are summarized in Table 6-1.

Measurement of Weight	Significance of Findings
Infants (Birth to 20 Months)	
Undress completely (including diaper) and lay on a balanced infant scale. Protect the scale surface with a cloth or paper liner.	**Clinical Alert** Weight loss or failure to gain weight may be related to dehydration, acute infections, feeding disorders, malabsorption, chronic disease, diabetes, anorexia nervosa, cocaine use by mother in prenatal period, or acquired immune deficiency syndrome (AIDS). A loss of 10% on a growth
Young Children (20 Months to 5 Years)	
Undress except for underpants, and weigh on a standing scale.	

chart is indicative of severe weight loss. Excessive weight gain may be related to chronic renal, pulmonary, or cardiovascular disorders or to endocrine dysfunction.

Older Children (5 Years and Older)

Remove shoes. Weigh clothed, on a standing scale.

Establishing Height

Measurement of Height	Significance of Findings
Infants (Birth to 20 Months)	
Lay infant flat. Have parent hold infant's head as the infant's legs are extended and pushed *gently* toward the table. Measure the distance between marks made indicating heel tips (with toes pointing inward) and vertex of head. *Do not use a cloth tape* for measurement, because it may stretch.	**Clinical Alert** Although short stature is usually genetically predetermined, it may also indicate chronic heart or renal disease, growth hormone deficiency, or malnutrition.
Children (20 Months and Older)	
Have child, in stocking feet or bare feet, stand straight on a standard scale, and measure with the attached marker, to the nearest 0.1 cm (0.03 in).	

Assessment of Eating Practices

Assessment of eating practices requires sensitivity on the part of the nurse. Eating practices are highly personal and can be more

Table 6-1 Physical growth during infancy and childhood

Age	Weight	Height
Infants		
0 to 6 months	Average weekly gain 140-200 gm (5-7 oz) Birth weight doubles by 4-6 mo	Average monthly gain 2.5 cm (1 in)
6 to 18 months	Average weekly gain 85-140 gm (3-5 oz) Birth weight triples by 1 year	Average monthly gain 1.25 cm (0.5 in)
Toddler		
18 months to 3 years	Average yearly gain 2-3 kg (4.4-6.6 lb)	Height at 2 years approximately half of adult height
1-2 years		Average gain 12 cm (4.8 in)
2-3 years		Average gain 6-8 cm (2.4-3.2 in)

Preschool-Aged Child		
3 to 6 years	Average yearly gain 1.8-2.7 kg (4-6 lb)	Yearly gain 6-8 cm (2.4-3.2 in)
School-Aged Child		
6 to 12 years	Average yearly gain 1.8-2.7 kg (4-6 lb)	Yearly gain 5 cm (2 in)
Preadolescent/Adolescent		
Girl, 10 to 14 years	Average gain 17.5 kg (38.5 lb)	95% of adult height achieved by onset of menarche Average gain 20.5 cm (8.1 in)
Boy, 12 to 16 years	Average gain 23.7 kg (52.1 lb)	95% of adult height achieved by 15 years Average gain 27.5 cm (11 in)

accurately assessed once a rapport has been established. Guilt, apprehension, and a desire to give the "right" responses can alter the accuracy of the assessment.

Table 6-2 lists eating habits typical of various age groups.

General Assessment

- Is your child on a special diet?
- Describe your child's typical diet over 24 hours (foods, fluids, amounts, frequencies).
- Are there cultural or ethnic influences that affect your child's diet? How?
- Have you any concerns?

Assessment of Feeding Practices of Infants

- How much weight did you (mother) gain during pregnancy?
- What vitamin supplements does your infant receive?
- Does your infant have any problems with feeding (lethargy, poor sucking, regurgitation, colic, irritability, rash, diarrhea)?
- Breast-fed infants
  - How long does your infant feed at one time?
  - Do you alternate breasts?
  - How do you recognize that your infant is hungry? Full?
  - Describe your infant's elimination and sleeping patterns.
  - Have you concerns related to breast-feeding?
  - Describe your usual daily diet.
- Formula-fed infants
  - What type of formula is your infant on?
  - How do you prepare the formula?
  - What type of bottle does your infant take?
  - Do you prop or hold your infant while feeding?
  - Have you concerns related to bottle-feeding?

Assessment of Feeding Practices of Toddlers and Children

- What foods does your child prefer? Dislike?
- Does the child snack? If so, when? What foods are given as snacks?

Assessment of Feeding Practices of Adolescents

- What foods do you prefer? Dislike?
- What foods do you choose for a snack?

Table 6-2 Eating habits and concerns common to various age groups

Age Group	Eating Practices	Concerns Arising from Eating Practices
Infants 0 to 18 months	Formula or breast milk forms major part of diet for first 6 months and is generally recommended until 1 year. Solid foods assume greater importance in second 6 months of life. By 1 year, infant is able to eat all solid foods unless food intolerance develops.	Mothers may feed child in accordance with practices followed in their own upbringing. Early introduction of solid foods (before 5 or 6 months) may contribute to obesity or allergies. Colic, regurgitation, diarrhea, constipation, bottle mouth syndrome, and rashes are common concerns associated with infant feeding. Yellowish skin coloration may accompany persistent feeding of carrots. Excess milk intake in later infancy may lead to milk anemia.

Continued.

Table 6-2 Eating habits and concerns common to various age groups—cont'd

Age Group	Eating Practices	Concerns Arising from Eating Practices
Toddlers/Preschool-Aged Children 18 months to 6 years	Appetites tend to be erratic because of sporadic energy needs. Appetites of toddlers and preschoolers are smaller than those of infants because of slowed growth. Toddlers and preschoolers have definite likes and dislikes. Likes include foods such as yogurt, fruit drinks, fruit breads, and cookies that are easy to eat and to handle. Dislikes include casseroles, liver, and cooked vegetables. Food is often consumed "on the go." Children may go on "food jags," where one food is preferred for a few days. Variety is desirable, but not necessary so long as the child eats from all	Some children may snack their way through the day and rarely consume a regular meal. Mealtimes may become a battle between parents and toddlers over types and amounts of food eaten. Parents may express concern over toddlers' or preschoolers' diminished appetite.

	food groups during the course of a day.	
School-Aged Children 6 to 12 years	Children generally have a good appetite and like variety. Plain foods still preferred. Increasing numbers of activities compete with mealtimes. Television and peers influence food choices.	Parents may express concern over table manners.
Adolescents 12 years and older	Food habits include skipping meals (especially breakfast), fast foods, snacking, and unusual food choices. Adolescents consume increasingly larger amounts of alcohol at younger ages. Adolescent girls frequently are calorie conscious and may diet.	Alcohol may form substantial portion of caloric intake. Preoccupation with food and feelings of guilt may be indicative of eating disorders. Anorexia nervosa and bulimia are serious disorders related to obsession to lose weight.

Are you satisfied with the quantity and kinds of food you eat?
Have you tried to change your food intake? In what ways?
Have you started your menstrual periods (girls)? Are you taking an oral contraceptive?
How active are you in sports or fitness activities?

Assessment of Physical Signs of Nutrition or Malnutrition

Many of the assessments related to nutritional status can be combined with other areas of the physical assessment. Table 6-3 outlines the head-to-toe observations that provide information about a child's nutritional status.

Related Nursing Diagnoses

Activity intolerance: Related to fatigue; inadequate protein and calories; electrolyte imbalance.

Bowel elimination, alterations in: Constipation related to formula intake; excess intake of calcium; decreased intake of fiber.

Bowel elimination, alterations in: Diarrhea related to deficiency of niacin; excess vitamin C; food intolerances; excess consumption of fresh fruit or other high-fiber foods.

Cardiac output, alteration in: Related to excess intake of niacin, potassium; inadequate intake of magnesium, potassium.

Comfort, alteration in: Related to neurologic disturbances; constipation; diarrhea.

Fluid volume excess: Related to overfeeding.

Fluid volume deficit: Related to inadequate intake of fluids; excessive loss of fluids secondary to diarrhea or vomiting.

Growth and development, alterations in: Related to excess of protein and calories; deficit of protein and calories; genetic endowment.

Health maintenance, alterations in: Related to lack of knowledge; alcohol abuse; skin lesions; dental caries; obesity; anorexia; bowel irregularity.

Knowledge deficit: Related to management of an age-appropriate diet.

Table 6-3 Physical assessment of nutrition

Body Area	Signs of Adequate/Appropriate Nutrition	Signs of Inadequate/Inappropriate Nutrition	Possible Causes of Inadequate/Inappropriate Nutrition
General growth	Height, weight, head circumference within 5th and 95th percentiles	Height, weight, head circumference below or above 5th and 95th percentiles	Protein, fats, vitamin A, niacin, calcium, iodine, manganese, zinc deficiency/excess
	Sexual development age appropriate	Delayed sexual maturation	Less than expected growth possibly related to disease (especially endocrine dysfunction) or to genetic endowment
			Vitamin A or D excess
Skin	Elastic, firm slightly dry; no lesions, rashes, hyperpigmentation	Dryness	Vitamin A deficiency
			Essential and unsaturated fatty acid deficiency
		Swollen red pigmentation (pellagrous dermatosis)	Niacin deficiency
		Hyperpigmentation	Vitamin B_{12}, folic acid, niacin deficiency

Continued.

Table 6-3 Physical assessment of nutrition—cont'd

Body Area	Signs of Adequate/Appropriate Nutrition	Signs of Inadequate/Inappropriate Nutrition	Possible Causes of Inadequate/Inappropriate Nutrition
Skin—cont'd		Edema	Protein deficiency or sodium excess
		Poor skin turgor	Water, sodium deficiency
		Petechiae	Ascorbic acid deficiency
		Delayed wound healing	Vitamin C deficiency
		Decreased subcutaneous tissue	Prolonged caloric deficiency
		Pallor	Iron, vitamin B_{12} or C, folic acid, pyridoxine deficiency
Hair	Shiny, firm, elastic	Dull, dry, thin, brittle, sparse, easily plucked	Protein, caloric deficiency
Head	Head evenly molded, with occipital prominence; facial features symmetric	Skull flattened, frontal bones prominent	Vitamin D deficiency
	Sutures fused by 12 to 18 months	Suture fusion delayed	Vitamin D deficiency
		Hard, tender lumps in occipital region	Vitamin A excess

Neck	Thyroid gland not obvious to inspection, palpable in midline	Thyroid gland enlarged, obvious to inspection	Iodine deficiency
Eyes	Clear, bright, shiny	Dull, soft cornea; white or gray spots on cornea (Bitot's spots)	Vitamin A deficiency
	Membranes pink and moist	Pale membranes	Iron deficiency
		Burning, itching, photophobia	Riboflavin deficiency
	Night vision adequate	Nightblindness	Vitamin A deficiency
		Redness, fissuring at corners of eyes	Riboflavin, niacin deficiency
Nose	Smooth, intact nasal angle	Cracks, irritation at nasal angle	Niacin deficiency, vitamin A excess
Lips	Smooth, moist, no edema	Angular fissures, redness and edema	Riboflavin deficiency, vitamin A excess
Tongue	Deep pink, papillae visible, moist, taste sensation, no edema	Paleness	Iron deficiency
		Red, swollen, raw	Folic acid, niacin, vitamin B or B_{12} deficiency
		Magenta coloration	Riboflavin deficiency
		Diminished taste	Zinc deficiency

Continued.

Table 6-3 Physical assessment of nutrition—cont'd

Body Area	Signs of Adequate/Appropriate Nutrition	Signs of Inadequate/Inappropriate Nutrition	Possible Causes of Inadequate/Inappropriate Nutrition
Gums	Firm, coral color	Spongy, bleed easily, receding	Ascorbic acid deficiency
Teeth	White, smooth, free of spots or pits	Mottled enamel, brown spots, pits,	Fluoride excess, or discoloration from antibiotics
		Defective enamel	Vitamin A, C, or D, or calcium, phosphorus deficiency
		Caries	Carbohydrate excess, poor hygiene
Cardiovascular system	Pulse and blood pressure within normal limits for age	Palpitations	Thiamin deficiency
		Rapid pulse	Potassium deficiency
		Arrhythmia	Niacin, potassium excess; magnesium, potassium deficiency
		High blood pressure	Sodium excess
Gastrointestinal system	Bowel habits normal for age	Constipation	Calcium excess, overrigid toilet training, inadequate

			intake of high fiber foods or fluids
		Diarrhea	Niacin deficiency; vitamin C excess; high consumption of fresh fruit, other high-fiber foods
Musculoskeletal system	Muscles firm and well developed, joints flexible and pain free, extremities symmetric and straight, spinal nerves normal	Muscles atrophied, dependent edema	Protein, caloric deficiency
		Knock-knee, bowleg, epiphyseal enlargement	Vitamin D deficiency; disease processes
		Bleeding into joints, pain	Vitamin C deficiency
		Beading on ribs	Vitamins C and D deficiency
Neurologic system	Behavior alert and responsive, intact muscle innervation	Listlessness, irritability, lethargy	Thiamine, niacin, pyridoxine, iron, protein, caloric deficiency
		Tetany	Magnesium deficiency
		Convulsions	Thiamine, pyridoxine, vitamin D, calcium deficiency; phosphorus excess
		Unsteadiness, numbness in hands and feet	Pyridoxine excess
		Diminished reflexes	Thiamine deficiency

Nutrition, alterations in: Less than body requirements related to lack of knowledge of adequate nutrition; crash or fad diets; anorexia; nausea and vomiting; allergy; congenital anomalies; growth spurts; inability to procure food.

Nutrition, alterations in: More than body requirements related to lack of basic nutritional knowledge; ethnic or family values.

Self-concept, disturbance in: Body image and self-esteem related to obesity.

Sensory-perceptual alterations: Related to fluid and electrolyte imbalance; alcohol abuse.

Sexual dysfunction: Secondary to obesity; alcohol abuse.

PART

MEASUREMENT OF VITAL SIGNS II

7 Body Temperature, Pulse, and Respirations

Nursing fundamentals textbooks provide comprehensive discussions of measurement of vital signs. Only significant pediatric variations in the measurement of temperature, pulse, and respirations are presented here.

Measurement of Body Temperature

Rationale

Environmental factors and relatively minor infections can produce a much higher temperature in infants and young children than would be expected in older children and adults. In very young infants, fever may be one of the few signs of an underlying disorder. In toddlers, febrile convulsions can parallel fever and are of particular concern. The absence or presence of fever and the cause of fever are important in planning nursing care. Body temperature should be measured on admission to the health care facility, before and after surgery or invasive diagnostic procedures, during the course of an unidentified infection, after fever reduction measures have been taken, and any time that an infant or child looks flushed, feels warm, or is lethargic.

Anatomy and Physiology

The temperature-regulating mechanisms in infants and young children are not well developed, and dramatic fluctuations can occur. A young child's temperature may vary as much as 1.6° C

Table 7-1 Body temperature in well children

Age	Temperature °C	°F
3 mo	37.5	99.4
1 yr	37.7	99.7
3 yr	37.2	99.0
5 yr	37.0	98.6
7 yr	36.8	98.3
9 yr	36.7	98.1
13 yr	36.6	97.8

Modified from Lowrey GH: Growth and development of children, ed 7, St Louis, 1978, Mosby–Year Book.

(3° F) in a single day. Fluctuations are less apparent as temperature-regulating mechanisms mature.

The control of body heat loss increases with age. The ability of muscles to shiver increases with maturity, and the child will accumulate ever greater amounts of adipose tissue necessary for insulation against heat loss. Heat production decreases with age. The infant produces relatively more heat per unit of body weight than the adult does, as reflected by the infant's higher average body temperature (Table 7-1). A variety of other factors also affect the body temperature of the child (Table 7-2).

Preparation

Ask the parent or child if the child has been febrile, and if so, whether the fever has followed a pattern. Sustained fevers show little fluctuation and are found in children with scarlet fever or central nervous system disorders. Intermittent fevers, with wide variations in body temperature, occur with bacteremia or viremia. Recurrent fevers occur with Hodgkin's disease.

Establish whether the parent has administered fever reduction measures, and if so, how recently. Ask whether the child has had recent surgery, been in contact with persons with infectious or communicable diseases, or been immunized recently. If the child is a young infant, ask whether the infant has been anorexic or irritable (more obvious signs of fever such as shivering and diaphoresis are not usually seen in the young infant). If the child is

Table 7-2 Factors influencing body temperature

Factor	Effect
Active exercise	May temporarily raise temperature
Stress, crying	Raises body temperature
Diurnal variation	Body temperature is lowest between 0100 and 0400 hours (1:00 and 4:00 AM), highest between 1600 and 1800 hours (4:00 and 6:00 PM)
Environment, including clothing	Body temperature can vary with room temperature, amount and type of clothing

5 years or older, assess the child's ability to understand and to follow directions, because oral temperature measurement may be desirable. If rectal temperature measurement is selected, the procedure may be left until near the end of the health assessment, because preschoolers, in particular, find it intrusive.

Guidelines for Measurement of Body Temperature

- Select the site for temperature measurement based on the child's age and condition (Table 7-3), and institutional policy.
- Position the child appropriately.
  - For axillary temperature, hold the child quietly on your lap. Diversions such as reading are useful.
  - For oral temperature, have the child sit or lie quietly.
  - For rectal temperature, younger infants can be placed in a supine position, with knees flexed toward the abdomen. Larger infants and children can be placed in prone or side-lying positions. If the parent is available, the child can wrap arms around the parent's neck and legs around the parent's waist.
- Always record the route by which the temperature was taken, because the differences between routes cannot be assumed as constant.
- In addition to measurement of body temperature, all children should be assessed for:
  - Signs and symptoms of dehydration, including poor skin turgor, dry mucous membranes, decreased or absent tearing

Table 7-3 Guidelines for selection of site for body temperature measurement

Site	Age Group	Contraindications
Axilla	All age groups, but particularly preschoolers, who tend to fear invasive procedures.	May be contraindicated when accuracy is especially critical or in initial stages of a fever, when axilla may not be sensitive to early changes.
Oral	Cooperative 5- and 6-year-old children, school-aged children, adolescents.	Do not use if the child is uncooperative or unable to follow directions, is comatose or seizure prone, has had oral surgery, mouth breathes, or is on oxygen.
Rectal	All age groups. Some sources recommend usage for children older than 2 years because of risks of breakage and perforation.	Do not use if the child has had anal surgery or has diarrhea or rectal irritation, or if it is possible to use oral or axillary sites. Presence of stool may decrease accuracy.
Tympanic	All age groups, but particularly toddlers and preschoolers who protest restraint and yet are unable to fully cooperate.	May be contraindicated in children with acute otitis media or sinusitus or children with very small external ear canals.

(in child older than 6 weeks of age), sunken eye orbits, dry body creases, and sunken fontanels (infants).
Flushed appearance.
Chills, as evidenced by shivering and piloerection.
Restlessness.
Lethargy.
Increased pulse and respiratory rates.
Twitching.

Related Nursing Diagnoses

Anxiety: Related to febrile seizures.

Body temperature, actual alteration in: Related to infection; inflammation; stress; dehydration; tumor; immunization.

Fluid volume deficit: Related to fever; increased metabolic rate; hyperpnea.

Knowledge deficit: Related to management of seizures; fever management techniques; recognition of signs and symptoms of fever.

Thermoregulation, ineffective: Related to immaturity of body systems.

Measurement of Pulse

Rationale

The measurement of pulse is a routine part of hospital procedure but should not be underestimated as an easily accessible indicator of the status of the cardiovascular system. Disorders of the cardiovascular system, the effects of fever, and the effects of drug therapies can be monitored through assessment of pulse. The pulse should be routinely monitored during disease processes, during fever, before and after surgery, and whenever a child's condition deteriorates.

Anatomy and Physiology

Approximately 8.5% of the body weight in the neonate is blood volume, compared with 7% to 7.5% in the older child and adult. The heart size increases as the child grows, with a resultant decrease in heart rate. Variations in heart rate are much more dramatic in the child than in the adult. Table 7-4 lists normal pulse

Table 7-4 Pulse rates in children at rest

Age	Average Rate	2 SD
Birth	140	50
1 mo	130	45
1-6 mo	130	45
6-12 mo	115	40
1-2 yr	110	40
2-4 yr	105	35
6-10 yr	95	30
10-14 yr	85	30
14-18 yr	82	25

From Lowrey GH: Growth and development of children, ed 7, St Louis, 1978, Mosby–Year Book.

Table 7-5 Influences on pulse rate

Influence	Effect
Medications	Aminophylline, racemic epinephrine, atropine sulfate increase pulse rate. Digoxin decreases pulse rate.
Activity	Activity increases pulse rate. Sustained, regular exercise eventually decreases rate. Pulse varies if a child is sleeping, increasing during inspiration, and decreasing during expiration (sinus arrhythmia). Crying and feeding increases pulse rate in an infant.
Hypoxia	Increases pulse rate.
Fever	Increases pulse rate by about 10 to 15 beats per °C temperature increase. High fever accompanied by low pulse and respiratory rate may signal a drug reaction. Low fever with high pulse and respiratory rates may signal septic shock.
Apprehension, acute pain	Increases pulse rate.
Hemorrhage	Increases pulse rate.

rates; Table 7-5, influences on pulse rate; and Table 7-6, deviations from normal pulse patterns.

Preparation

Ask the parent or child about a family history of arrhythmias, atherosclerosis, or myocardial infarction. Ask if the child has known heart disease or has experienced or is experiencing palpitations or arrhythmias. Determine if fever is present, and if the child has received medication recently.

Guidelines for Measurement of Pulse

- Measure the pulse when the infant or child is quiet. Because of lability of the pulse, carefully document the child's activity or anxiety level when the pulse is recorded.

Table 7-6 Deviations from normal pulse patterns

Pulse	Characteristics and Significance
Bradycardia	Slowed pulse rate.
Tachycardia	Increased pulse rate. An absence of apprehension, crying, increased activity, or fever, may indicate cardiac disease.
Sinus arrhythmia	Pulse rate increases during inspiration, decreases during expiration. Sinus arrhythmia is a normal variation in children, especially during sleep.
Alternating pulse (pulsus alternans)	Alteration of weak and strong beats. May indicate heart failure.
Bigeminal pulse	Coupled beats related to premature beats.
Paradoxical pulse	Strength of pulse diminishes with inspiration.
Thready pulse	Weak, rapid pulse. May be indicative of shock. Pulse is difficult to palpate; seems to appear and disappear.
Corrigan's pulse (water-hammer pulse)	Forceful, jerky beat caused by wide variation in pulse pressure.

- Select the appropriate site. The apical pulse is measured in children younger than 2 years of age, because the radial pulse is difficult to locate. The apical pulse should be measured at any age when the radial pulse is difficult to locate, when cardiac disease has been identified, or when the radial pulse is irregular.
- Listen for the apical pulse at the point of maximum impulse (PMI). This will be found in the *fourth intercostal space* in children *younger than 7 years*. In children *older than 7 years* the apical pulse will be found in the *fifth interspace*, and will be more lateral.
- Auscultate radial and apical pulses for 1 full minute.

Related Nursing Diagnoses

Anxiety: Related to pulse arrhythmias or irregularities.

Cardiac output, alterations in: Decreased, related to bradycardia; tachycardia; hypothermia or hyperthermia; surgery; medications; congenital heart defects; shock.

Fluid volume deficit: Related to hemorrhage.

Tissue perfusion, alteration in: Secondary to decreased cardiac output.

Measurement of Respirations

Rationale

Assessment of respiration involves external assessment of ventilation. Inasmuch as the quality and rate of respirations can be affected by disorders in every body system, the character of respirations must be carefully assessed and reported.

Anatomy and Physiology

Infants and young children inhale a relatively small amount of air, and exhale a relatively large amount of oxygen. Young children and infants have fewer alveoli and therefore less alveolar surface through which gas exchange can occur. These factors, together with a higher metabolic rate, are influential in increasing respiratory rates in infants and children. Table 7-7 outlines normal respiratory rates; and Table 7-8, influences on respiratory rates.

Table 7-7 Variations in respiration with age

Age	Rate (breaths/min)
Premature infant	40-90
Neonate	30-80
1 yr	20-40
2 yr	20-30
3 yr	20-30
5 yr	20-25
10 yr	17-22
15 yr	15-20
20 yr	15-20

From Lowrey GN: Growth and development of children, ed 7, St Louis, 1978, Mosby–Year Book.

Table 7-8 Influences on respiration

Influencing Factor	Effect
Age	Respiratory rate decreases as the child grows older. The rate tends to increase dramatically in infants and young children relative to anxiety, crying, fever, disease. The rhythm is irregular in young infants, who experience sharp increases in rate, and apneic spells. (Apneic spells of 15-20 seconds or longer are considered pathologic.)
Medications	Narcotic analgesics decrease respiratory rate. Xanthine derivatives may cause an increase in rate.
Position	Slumping impedes ventilatory movements.
Fever	Respirations increase in rate and depth.
Increased activity	Respirations increase in rate or depth.
Anxiety or fear	Respirations increase in rate and depth.
Pathologic states	Respiratory rate, rhythm, and depth alter as a result of cerebral trauma, respiratory disorders, hemorrhage, anemia, meningitis, cardiac disorders, infectious disorders, and tetanus.

Preparation

Ask the parent or child about the use of medications; whether there is difficulty breathing, or apnea (infants); and about the presence of respiratory infections. Inquire about a family history of cardiac or respiratory disorders.

Guidelines for Measurement of Respirations

- Assess the infant's or child's respirations before beginning more intrusive procedures. If the infant or child is already crying, wait for calmer behavior before assessing respiratory rates.
- Avoid letting the child know that respirations are being counted; self-consciousness may alter the respiratory rate and depth. Assess the respirations when counting the pulse or performing an assessment of the thorax and lungs.
- When assessing the respirations of *infants and younger children,* the nurse places fingers or a hand just below the child's xiphoid process so that the inspiratory rises can be felt. Alternatively, the respirations can be assessed by listening to breath sounds through the stethoscope.
- Observe a complete respiratory cycle (inspiration plus expiration).

  Count respirations for *1 full minute*. Respirations of infants and young children can be quite irregular.

  While counting, note the depth and rhythm of breathing. Depth is a subjective estimation, and is usually noted as shallow, normal, or deep. If unable to label a rhythm, describe it. Table 7-9 gives a description of respiratory rhythms.
- Observe the child for:

  Cyanosis of the nailbeds, indicative of *peripheral cyanosis*. Peripheral cyanosis may be caused by vasoconstriction, and is common in the young infant.

  Cyanosis of the lips and trunk, indicative of *central cyanosis*. Central cyanosis indicates a significant drop in the oxygen-carrying capacity of the blood.

  Restlessness, anxiety, and decreasing levels of consciousness, which can be related to hypoxia.

Table 7-9 Altered respiratory patterns

Pattern	Description
Dyspnea	Difficult or labored breathing; indicated by presence of retractions.
Bradypnea 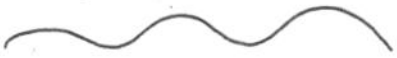	Abnormally slow rate of breathing; rhythm regular.
Tachypnea 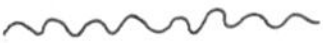	Abnormally fast rate of breathing.
Hyperpnea 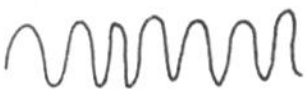	Rapid, deep respirations.
Apnea	Absence of respirations.
Cheyne-Stokes respiration (periodic breathing) 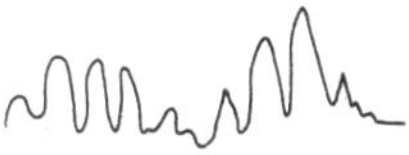	Periods of deep rapid breathing alternating with periods of apnea. Commonly seen in infants, and may be seen normally in children during deep sleep. Abnormal causes include drug-induced depression and brain damage.
Kussmaul's respiration 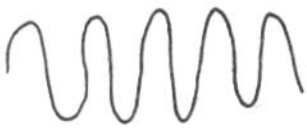	Abnormally deep breathing. May be rapid, normal, or slow. Commonly associated with metabolic acidosis.
Biot's respiration (ataxic breathing) 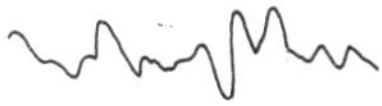	Unpredictable, irregular breathing. Seen with lower brain damage and respiratory depression.

Related Nursing Diagnoses

Activity intolerance: Related to inadequate oxygenation secondary to respiratory depression; ineffective respiratory effort.

Anxiety: Related to air hunger.

Breathing pattern ineffective: Related to obstruction; infection; medication; apnea; acidosis; brain damage.

Powerlessness: Related to inadequate oxygenation.

Blood Pressure 8

Rationale

Blood pressure readings provide significant information about the child's health status. Until recently, children younger than 3 years were commonly not screened for blood pressure, because of the extra skill and patience required to obtain a blood pressure reading in such young patients. The majority of children with hypertension have renal disease; many fewer have coarctation of the aorta or pheochromocytoma. Screening of blood pressure in young children permits early detection of serious disorders. Blood pressure determination is routine on admission to health care facilities and in postoperative procedures. It should also be performed after invasive diagnostic procedures and before and after administration of drugs known to alter blood pressure. Blood pressure is taken whenever a child "feels funny" or when a child's condition deteriorates.

Anatomy and Physiology

Blood pressure is a product of cardiac output and increased peripheral resistance. In the neonate, systolic blood pressure is low, reflecting the weaker ability of the left ventricle. As the child grows, the size of the heart and of the left ventricle also increases, resulting in steadily increasing blood pressure values. At adolescence the heart enlarges abruptly, which also results in an increase in blood pressure values, comparable to those of the adult (Table 8-1).

An increase in cardiac output or in peripheral resistance will raise blood pressure. Decrease in cardiac output or in peripheral resistance will lower blood pressure. Overall maintenance of blood pressure reflects an intimate relationship among cardiac

Table 8-1 Normal blood pressure values at various ages

Age	Systole/Diastole (mm Hg)
1 mo	86/54
6 mo	90/60
1 yr	96/65
2 yr	99/65
4 yr	99/65
6 yr	100/60
8 yr	105/60
10 yr	110/60
12 yr	115/60
14 yr	118/60
16 yr	120/65

Modified from Lowrey GH: Growth and development of children, ed 7, St Louis, 1978, Mosby–Year Book.

output, peripheral resistance, and blood volume, which can be influenced by a number of other factors (Table 8-2).

Equipment for Measuring Blood Pressure

- Pediatric stethoscope
- Sphygmomanometer with either a mercury or an aneroid manometer
- Ace or tensor bandage (flush technique)

Guidelines for Measurement of Blood Pressure

- Select appropriate method. Palpation rather than auscultation may be performed if the child has a narrow or deep brachial artery. The flush technique may be selected if it is impossible to obtain blood pressure readings in young children or infants by other means.
- Select appropriate site. Extremities in casts, those in which intravenous fluids are being infused, or those that are traumatized should not be used. Thighs may be selected if only large cuffs are available.
- Select appropriate cuff size. The cuff should cover no less than half and no more than two-thirds of the upper arm or thigh in

Table 8-2 Influences on blood pressure

Influence	Effect
Medications	Narcotic analgesics, general anaesthetics, diuretics decrease blood pressure. Aminophylline increases blood pressure.
Conditions	Blood pressure decreases during hemorrhage. Blood pressure increases with renal disease, increased intracranial pressure, coarctation of aorta (blood pressure in arms), pheochromocytoma, and acute pain. Pulse pressure widens with increased intracranial pressure.
Diurnal variation	Blood pressure usually is higher during morning and afternoon than during evening and night.
Apprehension and anxiety	Increases blood pressure.
Increased activity	Increases blood pressure.

children and adolescents (Table 8-3). An overly large cuff may produce low readings. A cuff that is too narrow may produce high readings. If a correctly fitting cuff is not available, a wider cuff may be used. (Wider cuffs do not create the low readings in infants and younger children that are produced in adults.) The cuff bladder should be long enough to encircle the arm without overlapping.

Table 8-3 Guidelines for selecting age-appropriate cuff sizes

	Width	
Age	cm	in
Infant	5-8	2-3
Child	9-10	3.5-3.75
Adult	12-13	4.75-5

- Check bulb and pressure valve. Valve should adjust smoothly.
- Check needle of aneroid manometer. It should be at zero.
- Check mercury column of mercury manometer. It should be at zero.
- Blood pressure readings should be performed before other anxiety-producing procedures. The infant or child should be sitting quietly or lying down. The very young child may be most comfortable cradled in the parent's arms or lap.

Preparation

Ask the parent or child about family history of hypertension or cardiac or kidney disease. Ask if the child has or has had headache, nose bleeds, swelling, or alterations in voiding patterns.

Auscultation Method of Blood Pressure Measurement

Assessment	Findings
Select appropriate site and cuff. Position the child's limb. The arm should be at heart level. If positioned below the heart, a falsely high reading may be obtained. If obtaining a thigh reading, the child may be positioned on the abdomen or with the knee slightly flexed. Expose the limb completely. Compression of the limb by rolled up clothing may give a low reading. If the child is upset by removal of clothing, it is best to apply the cuff over the sleeve rather than rolling it up. Rolling produces a tight band.	
Palpate the brachial artery if using the arm, or the popliteal artery if using the thigh. Ensure that the cuff is fully	Viewing the manometer from above or below gives inaccurate readings.

Assessment	Findings
deflated. Center the arrows on the cuff over the brachial artery of the arm, or position the bladder over the posterior aspect of the thigh. Position the manometer at eye level.	
Palpate the radial or popliteal artery, and inflate the cuff to 30 mm Hg above the point at which the pulse disappears.	
Deflate the cuff; wait 30 seconds.	Inadequate release of venous congestion gives falsely high readings.
Place the earpieces of the stethoscope in your ears. Earpieces should point forward to be inserted correctly.	Incorrect placement of earpieces produces muffling or no sound at all.
Relocate the brachial or the popliteal artery. Place the bell or the diaphragm over the artery. Turn the valve of the pressure bulb clockwise until tight, and inflate cuff to 30 mm Hg above the child's systolic reading.	Improper placement of the stethoscope produces low systolic and high diastolic readings.
Gradually release the valve to reduce pressure at a rate of 2 to 3 mm Hg/sec.	Rapid release may cause inaccurate reading of the systolic pressure.
Observe the point at which the first clear reading is obtained (systolic pressure) and at which the first muffling occurs (diastolic pressure).	In children younger than 1 year, thigh pressures should equal arm pressures; in children older than 1 year, thigh pressure is approximately 20 mm Hg higher. **Clinical Alert** A low thigh pressure reading may indicate coarctation of the aorta.

Assessment	Findings
Deflate the cuff rapidly once readings have been obtained. Wait 30 seconds before obtaining further readings.	**Clinical Alert** Repeat blood pressure readings if lower or higher than expected. Document and report persistently elevated or lowered blood pressure readings. Consistently elevated serial readings may be indicative of hypertension. Persistently low diastolic pressure may be indicative of a patent ductus arteriosus. *Pulse pressure* (difference between systolic and diastolic pressures) of more than 50 mm Hg may be indicative of congestive heart failure. Pulse pressure of less than 10 mm Hg may be indicative of aortic stenosis.

Palpation Method of Blood Pressure Measurement

Assessment	Findings
Select appropriate site and cuff. Position child's limb, and prepare the cuff as though determining blood pressure by auscultation method.	
Palpate the brachial or the radial artery (arm) or the popliteal artery (thigh), and inflate the cuff 30 mm Hg above point at which pulse disappears.	

Assessment	Findings
Slowly deflate the cuff, at a rate of 2 to 3 mm Hg/sec.	
Determine point at which the pulse is first felt. This is the *systolic* pressure. The diastolic pressure cannot be determined by this method.	The systolic pressure obtained by radial palpation is approximately 10 mm Hg lower than arm pressure.

Flush Method of Blood Pressure Measurement

Assessment	Findings
Wrap cuff around the limb. Elevate the limb. Wrap an elastic bandage from the fingers toward the antecubital space (or from the toes toward the knee).	
Inflate the cuff above the expected systolic pressure.	
Remove bandage. Place the child's arm at his or her side.	The limb will appear pale.
Slowly deflate the cuff until color suddenly returns. The reading is taken when color appears.	The value (flush pressure) obtained is the mean blood pressure (average of the diastolic and systolic pressures).

Related Nursing Diagnoses

Cardiac output, alteration in: Decreased, related to arrhythmias; congenital anomalies; medications.

Fluid volume, alteration in: Related to hemorrhage.

Tissue perfusion, alteration in: Related to hypotension.

PART

ASSESSMENT OF BODY SYSTEMS

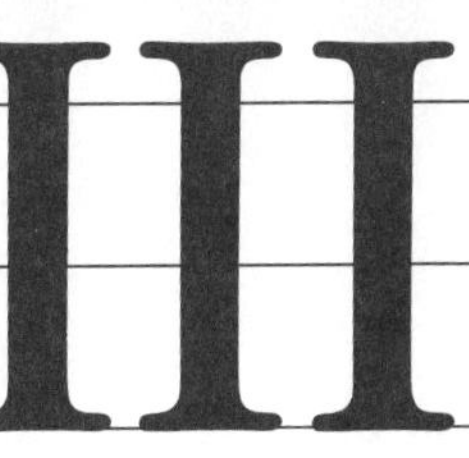

Integument 9

Assessment of the integument involves inspection and palpation of skin, nails, hair, and scalp and may be combined with assessment of other areas of the body.

Rationale

Assessment of the integument, or skin, should be an integral part of every health assessment, regardless of setting or situation. Many common pathophysiologic disorders have associated integumentary disorders. For example, many contagious childhood diseases have associated characteristic rashes. Rashes of all sorts are common in childhood. The integument yields much information about the physical care that a child receives and about the nutritional, circulatory, and hydration status of the child, which is valuable in planning health teaching interventions.

Anatomy and Physiology

The skin, which begins to develop during the eleventh week of gestation, consists of three layers (Figure 9-1). The *epidermis* is the outermost layer and is further divided into four layers. The top layer, or horny layer (stratum corneum), is of primary importance in protecting the internal homeostasis of the body. Melanin, produced by the regeneration layer of the epidermis, is the main pigment of the skin. The *dermis* underlies the epidermis and contains blood vessels, lymphatic vessels, hair follicles, and nerves. *Subcutaneous tissue* underlies the dermis and helps to cushion, contour, and insulate the body. This final layer contains sweat and sebaceous glands. The sebaceous glands produce sebum, which may have some bactericidal effect.

The skin has four main functions: protection against injury,

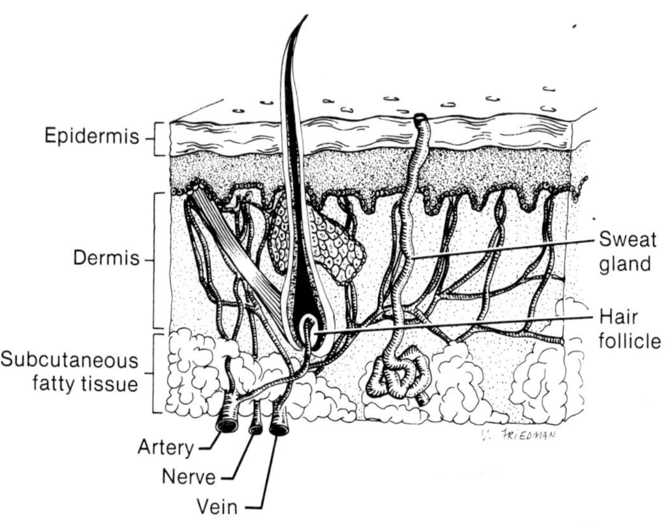

Figure 9-1
Normal skin layers.
(From Potter PA: Pocket nurse guide to physical assessment, St Louis, 1986, Mosby–Year Book.)

thermoregulation, impermeability, and sensor of touch, pain, heat, and cold.

The normal pH of the skin is acidic, which is thought to protect the skin from bacterial invasion. In infants the pH of the skin is higher, the skin is thinner, and the secretion of sweat and sebum is minimal. As a result, infants are more prone to skin infections and conditions than older children and adults. Further, because of loose attachment between the dermis and epidermis, infants and children tend to blister easily.

Preparation

Inquire about a family history of skin disorders, the life-style of the family, and recent changes in life-style. Ask when lesions began and whether other symptoms accompanied the lesions. Ask the parent to describe the size, configuration, distribution, type, and color of the lesions.

A well-illuminated room with white walls is essential for proper visualization of the skin. (Yellow walls may give the appearance of jaundice, and blue walls the appearance of cyanosis.) The room should also be warm.

Assessment of Skin

Assessment of the skin is usually performed during assessment of each body system.

Assessment	Findings
Observe the skin for odor.	**Clinical Alert** The presence of odor may indicate poor hygiene or infection.
Observe the color and pigmentation of the skin. If a color change is suspected, carefully inspect the areas of the body where there is less melanin (nailbeds, earlobes, sclerae, conjunctivae, lips, mouth). Inspect the abdomen (an area less exposed to sunlight) and the trunk. Use natural daylight for assessment if *jaundice* is suspected. Pressing a glass slide against a skin area produces blanching, which supplies contrast and enables closer assessment of the presence of jaundice. If a child has a different pigmentation from that of the accompanying parent, ask about the absent parent for hereditary trait recognition.	Overall skin color normally varies between and within races. For example, black children normally have a bluish tinge to gums and nailbeds. **Clinical Alert** A brown color to the skin may indicate Addison's disease or some pituitary tumors. A reddish blue skin tone suggests polycythemia. Red skin color may result from exposure to cold, hyperthermia, blushing, alcohol, or inflammation (if localized). Blue (cyanosis) coloration of nails may indicate *peripheral* or *central* cyanosis. Peripheral cyanosis may arise from anxiety or cold; central cyanosis is indicative of a marked drop in the oxygen-carrying capacity of the blood and also involves the *lips, mouth,* and *trunk.*

Assessment	Findings
	Yellow skin color may be indicative of jaundice (which accompanies liver disease, red cell hemolysis, biliary obstruction, or severe infection in infants), and is best observed in the sclerae, the mucous membranes, and on the abdomen.
	Yellowing of the palms, soles, and face (and not of the sclerae or mucous membranes) may indicate carotenemia, produced from ingestion of carrots, squash, and sweet potatoes.
	Yellowing of the exposed skin areas (and not of the sclerae and mucous membranes) may indicate chronic renal disease.
	Bruising in soft tissue areas (for example, buttocks) rather than on shins, knees, or elbows may be indicative of child abuse.
	A generalized lack of color involving the skin, hair, and eyes is indicative of albinism.
	Pallor (lack of pink tones in whites; ash gray color in blacks), suggestive of syncope, fever, shock, or anemia, is best observed in the face, mouth, conjunctivae, and nails.
Observe the moistness of exposed skin areas and mucous membranes.	The skin is normally slightly dry. Exposed areas normally feel dryer than body creases.

Assessment	Findings
Lightly stroke body creases. Compare body creases, one to another.	Mucous membranes should be moist. **Clinical Alert** Dry skin on the lips, hands, or genitalia is suggestive of contact dermatitis. Generalized dryness, accompanied by moist body creases and moist mucous membranes, is indicative of overexposure to the sun, overbathing, or poor nutrition. Dry arm creases and mucous membranes suggest dehydration. Clamminess may be indicative of shock or perspiration.
Palpate the skin with the back of the hand to determine *temperature*. Compare each side of the body with the other, and the upper with the lower extremities.	**Clinical Alert** Generalized hyperthermia may indicate fever, sunburn, or a brain disorder. Localized hyperthermia may indicate burn or infection. Generalized hypothermia may indicate shock. Local hypothermia may result from exposure to cold.
Inspect and palpate the texture of the skin. Note the presence of scars and excessive scar tissue (keloid).	An infant's or child's skin is normally smooth and even. **Clinical Alert** Rough, dry skin may indicate overbathing, poor nutrition, exposure to weather, or an endocrine disorder. Flaking or scaling between the fingers or toes may be related to eczema, dermatitis, or a fungal infection.

Assessment	Findings
	Oily scales on the scalp are indicative of seborrheic dermatitis (cradle cap). Hypopigmented, scaly patches on the face and upper body, or scattered papules (Table 9-1) over the arms, thighs, and buttocks, and fine, superficial scales may be indicative of eczema. A crackling sensation on palpation may be indicative of subcutaneous emphysema.
Palpate for *turgor* by grasping a fold on the upper arm or abdomen between the fingers and quickly releasing. Note the ease with which the skin moves (mobility) and returns to place (turgor) without residual marks.	Skin normally returns quickly to place with no residual marks. **Clinical Alert** A skinfold that returns slowly to place or retains marks commonly indicates dehydration or malnutrition. Other possible causes are chronic disease and muscle disorders.
Palpate for *edema* by pressing a thumb into areas that look swollen.	**Clinical Alert** Thumb indentations that remain after the thumb is removed are indicative of pitting edema. Edema in the periorbital areas may indicate crying, allergies, recent sleep, or renal disease. Edema (dependent) of the lower extremities and buttocks may indicate renal or cardiac disorders.

Assessment	Findings
Inspect and palpate the skin for *lesions* (Table 9-1). Note the distribution, shape, color, size, and consistency of the lesions and birthmarks (Table 9-3).	**Clinical Alert** Rashes are associated with a number of childhood disorders (Table 9-2).
	Petechiae and ecchymoses may indicate a bleeding tendency.
Enquire about pruritis.	

Text continues on p. 88.

Table 9-1 Common skin lesions

Lesion	Description
Primary Lesions (arise from normal skin)	
Macule 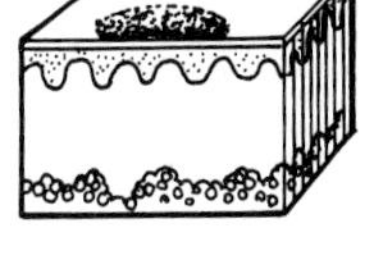	Small (less than 1 cm or 0.4 in) flat mass; differs from surrounding skin. Example: freckle.
Papule 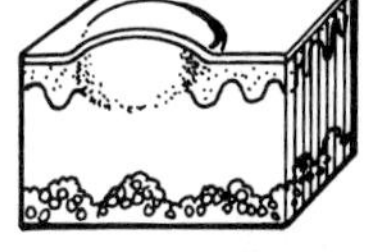	Small (less than 1 cm or 0.4 in) raised solid mass. Example: small nevus.
Nodule 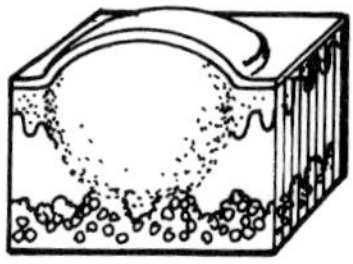	Solid, raised mass; slightly larger (1-2 cm or 0.4-0.8 in) and deeper than a papule.

Continued.

Table 9-1 Common skin lesions—cont'd

Lesion	Description
Tumor 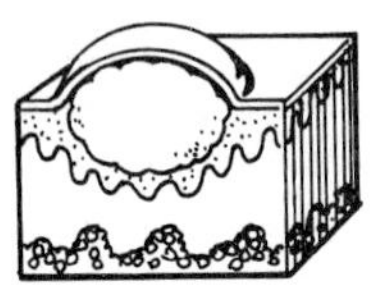	Solid, raised mass; larger than a nodule; may be hard or soft.
Wheal 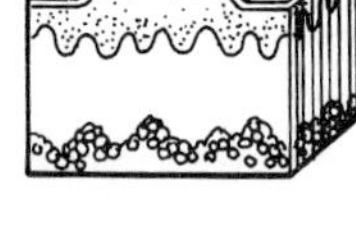	Irregularly shaped, transient area of skin edema. Example: hive, insect bite, allergic reaction.
Vesicle 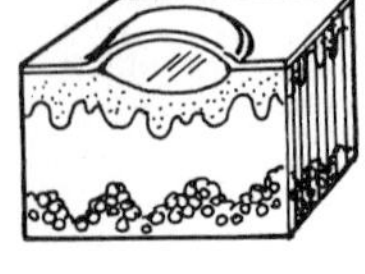	Small (less than 1 cm or 0.4 in) raised, fluid-filled mass. Example: herpes simplex, varicella.
Bulla 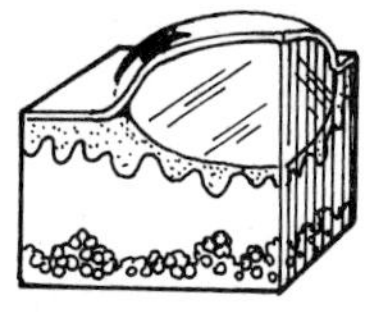	Raised fluid-filled mass; larger than a vesicle. Example: second-degree burn.
Pustule 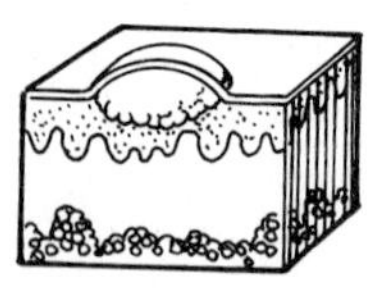	Vesicle containing purulent exudate. Example: acne, impetigo, staphylococcal infections.

Table 9-1 Common skin lesions—cont'd

Lesion	Description
Secondary Lesions (arise from changes in primary lesions)	
Scale 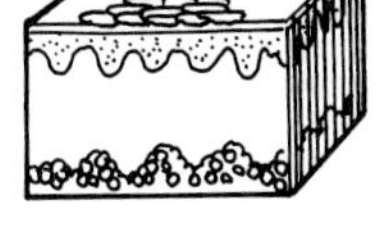	Thin flake of exfoliated epidermis. Example: psoriasis, dandruff.
Crust 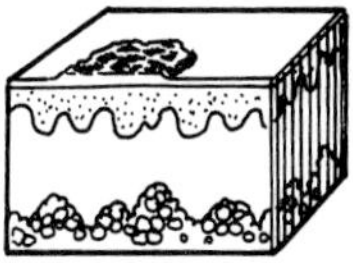 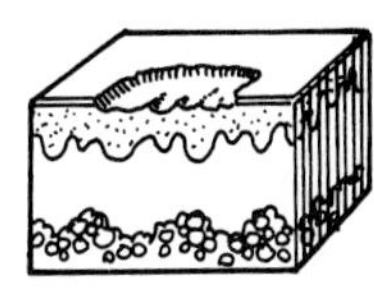	Dried residue of serum, blood, or purulent exudate. Example: eczema.
Erosion 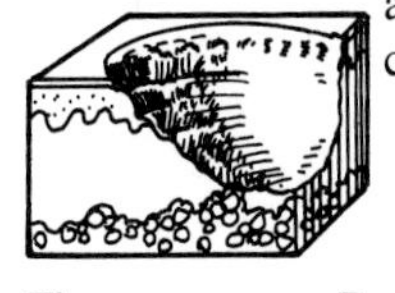	Moist lesion resulting from loss of superficial epidermis. Example: rupture of lesion in varicella.
Ulcer	Deep loss of skin surface; may extend to dermis and subcutaneous tissue. Example: syphilitic chancre, decubitus ulcer.
Fissure 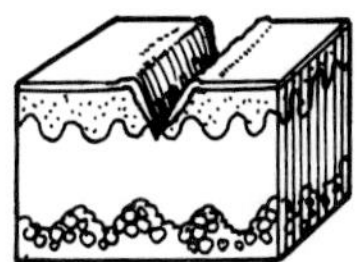	Deep, linear crack in skin. Example: athlete's foot.

Continued.

Table 9-1 Common skin lesions—cont'd

Lesion	Description
Lichenification 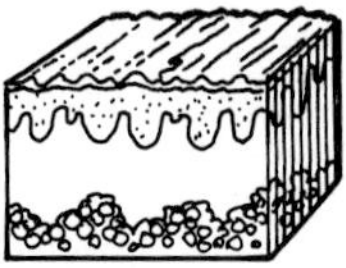	Thickened skin with accentuated skin furrows. Example: sequela of eczema.
Striae 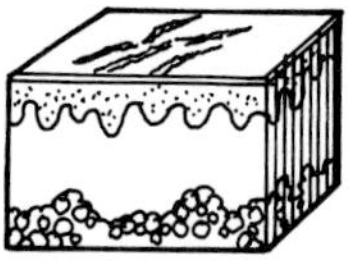	Thin white or purple stripes, commonly found on abdomen. May result from pregnancy or weight gain.
Purpuric Lesions	
Petechia 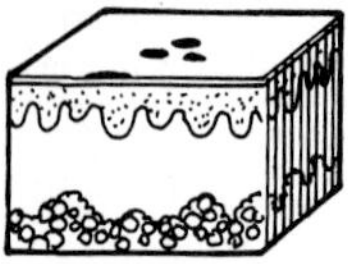	Flat, round, deep red or purplish mass (less than 3 mm or 0.1 in).
Ecchymosis 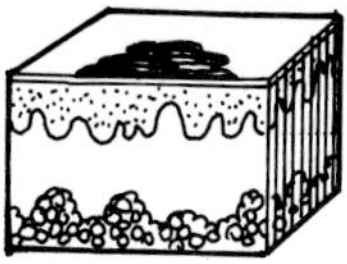	Mass of variable size and shape; initially purplish, fading to green, yellow, then brown.

Table 9-2 Distribution and characteristics of lesions associated with common childhood disorders

Disorder	Accompanying Lesions
Allergic Disorders	
Allergic reaction	Almost any type of lesion possible. Common manifestations are urticaria (hives), eczema, and contact dermatitis. Lesions may be intensely pruritic.
Urticaria	Wheals may be small or large, discrete or confluent, sparse or profuse. Wheals tend to come in crops, and fade in a few hours.
Eczema (atopic dermatitis)	Acute: erythema, vesicles, exudate, and crusts. Chronic: pruritic, dry, scaly, and thickened rash. Infantile form found on cheeks, forehead, scalp, and extensor surfaces. Childhood form found on wrists, ankles, and flexor surfaces.
Contact dermatitis	Pruritic red swelling that may be well demarcated from normal skin. Papules and bullae may be present.
Contagious Diseases	
Mumps	Painful swelling of parotid glands. May be unilateral or bilateral.
Measles (rubeola)	Red maculopapular rash that begins on face. Confluent at early sites of involvement, discrete at later sites. Becomes brownish in 3-4 days, and desquamates.
Rubella (German measles)	Pinkish red maculopapular rash that begins on face and spreads downward. Discrete lesions. Rash disappears within 3 days.
Roseola (baby measles)	Rose-pink macules or maculopapules that appear first on trunk before spreading. Discrete lesions fade on pressure. Nonpruritic. Rash disappears in 1-2 days.

Continued.

Table 9-2 Distribution and characteristics of lesions associated with common childhood disorders—cont'd

Disorder	Accompanying Lesions
Chickenpox (varicella zoster)	Rash progresses from macule to papule to vesicle to crust. Pruritic. Begins on trunk and spreads primarily to face and proximal extremities.
Scarlet fever	Tiny red lesions involve all but the face; more intense in joint areas. Desquamation begins in 1 week. Tongue initially is white and swollen (first 1-2 days), then becomes red and swollen.
Bacterial Infections	
Impetigo contagiosa	Rash begins with reddish macule, then vesicle appears. Vesicle ruptures, producing a moist erosion. Exudate dries, producing a honey-colored crust. Pruritic.
Cellutis	Skin red, swollen, warm to touch, firmly infiltrated. "Streaking" may be present.
Viral Infections	
Herpes simplex (cold sore)	Grouped vesicles on an erythematous base, found near lips, nose, genitalia, buttocks. Vesicles dry, leaving a crust.
Herpes zoster (shingles)	Rash follows dermatome of affected nerve, and appears in crops of vesicles. Pain and itching are common.
Fungi	
Tinea capitis	Pruritic circumscribed areas of scaling on the scalp. Alopecia present.

Table 9-2 Distribution and characteristics of lesions associated with common childhood disorders—cont'd

Disorder	Accompanying Lesions
Tinea corporis	Pruritic red, round or oval scaly areas. Central area clear.
Tinea pedis (athlete's foot)	Maceration and fissuring between toes, or vesicles on plantar surface. Pruritic.
Infestations	
Scabies	Linear, brownish gray burrows are produced by the female mite. Sarcoptic infestations produce papules, pustules, vesicles, and hives. In infants, lesions are primarily found on face, palms, and soles. In children, lesions are commonly found on apposed surfaces of skin and interdigital areas, on the extensor surfaces of joints and wrists, lower back, abdomen, genitalia, and buttocks.
Pediculosis corporis (body lice)	Lesions appear as red macules, wheals, excoriated papules, on the back and on areas that have close contact with clothing. Pruritic.
Miscellaneous	
Psoriasis	Thick, dry, red lesions covered with silvery scales. Lesions appear on scalp, ears, forehead, eyebrows, trunk, elbows, knees, and genitalia. More common in children 5 years of age and older.
Seborrheic dermatitis (cradle cap)	Oily, scaly patches on the scalp or along the hairline.

Table 9-3 Birthmarks and their description

Birthmark	Description
Vascular Nevi	
Salmon patch ("stork beak" mark)	Common. Flat, light pink mark found on the eyelids, in nasolabial region, or at the nape of the neck. Most disappear by the end of the first year of life.
Nevus flammeus (port-wine stain)	Flat, deep red or purplish red patches. Enlarge as child grows.
Strawberry nevus (raised hemangioma)	Begins as circumscribed grayish white area; becomes red, raised, well defined. May not be present at birth; resolves spontaneously by 9 years of age.
Hyperpigmented Nevi	
Mongolian spot	Large, flat, blue, black, or slate-colored area found on the buttocks and in the lumbosacral region.

Assessment of Nails

Assessment	Findings
Inspect nails for color, shape, and condition.	**Clinical Alert** Clubbing may indicate chronic respiratory or cardiac disease. Convex or concave curving nails may be hereditary or related to injury, iron deficiency, or infection.
Inspect nails for nail biting, skin picking, infection.	

Assessment of Hair

Assessment	Findings
Assess hair for distribution, color, texture, amount, and quality. Hair distribution is useful in estimating sexual maturity.	Hair normally covers all but the palms, soles, inner labial surfaces (girls), and prepuce and glans penis (boys). Scalp hair is normally, shiny, silky, strong. **Clinical Alert** Dry, brittle, or depigmented hair may indicate nutritional deficiency. A hairline that extends to mid-forehead may be normal or may indicate cretinism. Alopecia (loss of hair) may be related to tinea capitis, hair pulling, or persistent positioning on one side. Hair tufts on the spine or buttocks may indicate spina bifida. White eggs that are firmly attached to hair shafts are indicative of head lice.

Related Nursing Diagnoses

Comfort, alteration in: Related to pruritis; loss of skin surface.

Hyperthermia: Secondary to infection.

Knowledge deficit: Related to hygienic needs; prevention of infection.

Infection, high risk for: Related to loss of skin integrity.

Oral mucous membrane, alterations in: Secondary to infection; dehydration.

Parenting, high risk for or actual alteration in: Related to inappropriate caretaking behaviors.

Self-concept, disturbance in body image, self-esteem: Secondary to presence of acne, birthmarks, infectious lesions.

Skin integrity, impairment of: Related to injury, infection, nutritional disorders.

Tissue integrity, impaired: Related to injury; infection; altered nutritional state; altered pigmentation; developmental factors; alterations in turgor.

Head and Neck

10

Assessment of the neck includes evaluation of the trachea and the thyroid gland. The head is assessed for size, shape, and symmetry. The fontanels and sutures are examined, and head control is noted. Proceeding downward from the head to the neck provides a smooth progression of assessment.

Rationale

Examination of the head and neck is important in screening pediatric clients for acute disorders and long-term disabilities. The determination of disorders such as skull asymmetry can also signal the need for parent teaching.

Anatomy and Physiology

The head accounts for one fourth of the body length and one third of the body weight in the newborn infant, in comparison with one eighth of the body length and one tenth of the body weight in the adult. Head size, which is 32 to 38 cm (12.5 to 14 in) at birth, normally exceeds chest circumference by 1 to 2 cm (0.4 to 0.8 in) until 18 months of age. After 18 months, chest growth exceeds head size by 5 to 7 cm (2 to 2.75 in) (see Appendix B for charts of head circumference norms). The newborn skull consists of separate bones that fuse when brain growth is complete. Soft fibrous tissue joints, called sutures, separate the bones (Figure 10-1). These sutures, which can be felt as prominent ridges, begin to unite by 6 months of age, but may be separated by increased intracranial pressure until 12 years of age.

Fontanels are formed by the juncture of three or more skull bones (Figure 10-1) and are felt as soft concavities. Normally only the posterior and anterior fontanels can be palpated. The

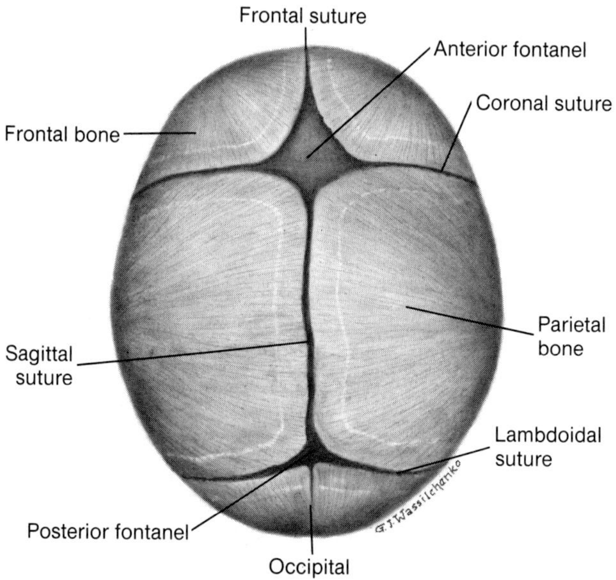

Figure 10-1
Location of sutures and fontanels.
(From Whaley LJ, Wong DL: Nursing care of infants and children, ed 4, St Louis, 1991, Mosby–Year Book.)

posterior fontanel may be closed at birth, and should always be closed by the second month. The anterior fontanel closes between 9 and 18 months of age.

By 4 months of age the infant should be able to hold the head erect and in midline. By 6 months no significant head lag should be noted when the child is pulled to a sitting position.

The neck in the infant and toddler is short, but by 4 years of age it assumes adult proportions. Although fully active at birth, the thyroid gland may not be palpable in infants and young children.

Preparation

Sit or lay the child in a comfortable position. The infant or young child may be most at ease on the mother's lap.

Equipment for Measurement of Head Circumference

Paper or narrow flexible metal tape (Do not use cloth tape, because it may stretch.)

Measurement	Findings
Measure head circumference if the child is 2 years of age or younger or if the size of child's head warrants concern. Place the tape around the head at points just above the eyebrows and the pinna and around the occipital prominence (Figure 10-2). If head circumference is measured daily, the head should be marked at key points to ensure consistency of measurement.	**Clinical Alert** If an infant's head circumference is above or below growth norms or the infant's established percentile, further evaluation is indicated. An abnormally large head circumference may indicate hydrocephalus. A small head circumference may indicate craniostenosis or microcephaly. Infants born to mothers who use cocaine may have smaller head circumferences.

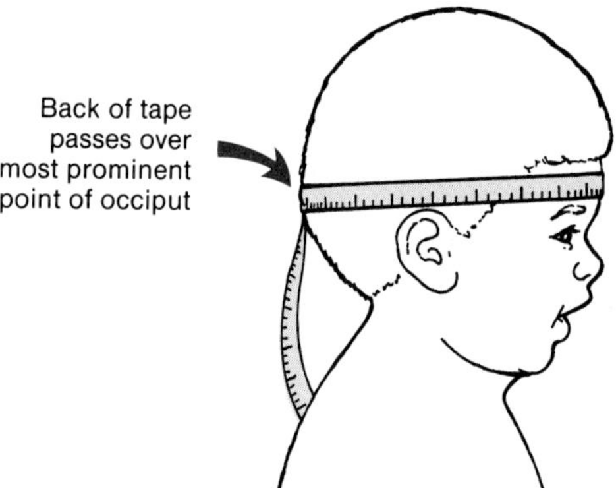

Figure 10-2
Measurement of head circumference.

Assessment of Head

Assessment	Findings
Observe the shape and symmetry of the infant's head from different angles. If possible, also note the shape and symmetry of the parents' heads.	Minor asymmetry in infants younger than 4 months is common and is related to molding. A head may be longer, narrower, or flatter than expected, as a result of genetic influences. **Clinical Alert** A markedly flattened occiput may be the result of persistent placement of the child in the supine position. If flattening is observed, ask the parents about the child's preferred sleep or play position. Parent teaching may be indicated. Head asymmetry may reflect premature closure of suture lines and requires further evaluation.
Palpate the suture lines in infants.	Sutures are felt as prominent ridges. In a newborn infant the suture lines override as a result of molding, but usually flatten by 6 months.
Observe and palpate the fontanels, if open, while the infant is sitting.	The anterior fontanel should be soft, flat, and pulsatile. The fontanel bulges slightly when the infant is crying. **Clinical Alert** A bulging fontanel may indicate increased intracranial pressure and is found in conditions such as head injury, meningitis, or neoplasm.

Assessment	Findings
	A depressed fontanel may indicate dehydration.
Measure the width and length of an open anterior fontanel.	Until 9 to 12 months the anterior fontanel measures from 1 to 5 cm (0.4 to 2 in) in length and width. **Clinical Alert** An abnormally small or large fontanel may suggest a bone growth disorder.

Related Nursing Diagnoses

Comfort, alteration in: Pain related to increased intracranial pressure.

Coping, ineffective family: Related to physical handicap; mental handicap secondary to congenital defects or altered brain pressures.

Family processes, alteration in: Related to nature of the condition; uncertain future.

Fear or anxiety: Related to implications of the condition; uncertain future.

Fluid volume deficit: Related to nausea and vomiting; difficulty in swallowing.

Growth and development, altered: Related to physical handicap; mental handicap.

Knowledge deficit: Related to positioning.

Mobility, impaired: Related to sensorimotor impairment.

Self-care deficit: Related to inability or difficulty in performing age-appropriate activities of daily living; secondary to sensorimotor impairment.

Self-concept, disturbance in: Related to physical deformity; interruption or failure in achieving developmental tasks.

Assessment of Neck

Assessment	Findings
Pull the infant to a sitting position while observing head control.	The infant younger than 4 months may show some head lag when pulled to a sitting position. **Clinical Alert** Significant head lag after 6 months may indicate cerebral palsy.
Put the child's head and neck through a full range of motion. The older child may be asked to look up, down, and sideways.	The child should exhibit no pain or limitation of movement in any direction. **Clinical Alert** Pain and resistance to flexion may indicate meningeal irritation. Lateral resistance to motion may indicate torticollis as a result of injury to the sternocleidomastoid muscle.
Inspect the neck for swelling, webbing, extra folds of skin, and vein distention.	**Clinical Alert** Webbing and extra neck folds may indicate Turner's syndrome. Swelling of the neck may indicate mumps or throat or mouth infection. Vein distention may be present with labored respirations.
Palpate the trachea by placing the thumb on one of the trachea and the index finger on the other. Slide the fingers up and down while the child's neck is slightly hyperextended.	The trachea should be at midline or slightly to the right. **Clinical Alert** Any shift in the position of the trachea should be noted, as serious lung problems may be present.

Assessment	Findings
Palpate the thyroid gland by standing behind the child and placing your fingers or hands gently over the area of the gland (at the base of the neck). The gland rises as a mass as the child swallows. Palpation of the thyroid gland in the infant and young child is difficult because of the shortness of the neck. Infants are best examined while lying supine across a parent's lap.	In normal children the thyroid gland may not be felt.

Related Nursing Diagnoses

Comfort, alteration in: Pain secondary to infection; meningeal irritation.

Coping, ineffective family: Related to situational crisis.

Fear: Related to rapid onset of illness.

Hyperthermia: Related to altered metabolic rates secondary to altered thyroid function.

Hypothermia: Related to altered metabolic rates secondary to altered thyroid function.

Mobility, impaired: Related to neuromuscular deficits.

Self-care deficit: Related to inability or interruption in performing age-appropriate activities of daily living.

Swallowing, impaired: Secondary to enlarged thyroid gland; altered level of consciousness.

Ears

11

Assessment of the ears involves inspection of the external and internal ear, testing of hearing acuity, and otoscopic examination. The nurse also focuses on the child's health history in an effort to identify factors that could place the child at risk for hearing problems.

Rationale

Ear disorders are disruptive to language, speech, and social development. Early screening and detection can assist in minimizing or eliminating hearing deficiencies and their effects. Temporary and correctable conditions such as otitis media are common in young children but may go undetected. Abnormalities of the external ear can be important in alerting health professionals to the presence of syndromes and should be reported. Assessment of the ear is performed in conjunction with the eye examination, because eye problems are nearly twice as common in children with hearing deficiencies.

Anatomy and Physiology

The ear consists of the external ear, the middle ear, and the inner ear. The outer ear consists of the auricle, the cartilaginous shell, and the external ear canal. In children younger than 3 years the canal points upward; in older children it is directed downward and forward. The lining of the external ear canal secretes cerumen, which protects the ear.

The middle ear consists of the tympanum (eardrum) and three bones (ossicles) that touch the tympanum on one side and the membrane covering the opening to the inner ear on the other side. Vibrations of the tympanum are transmitted through the ossicles to the inner ear. The middle ear also contains an opening to the eustachian tube. The eustachian tube allows secretions to pass from the middle ear to the nasopharnyx and enables air to enter the middle ear from the throat. Equalization of air pressure between the external ear canal and middle ear is essential for proper functioning of the tympanic membrane. The shorter and less angled eustachian tube in infants and young children permits secretions from the nose and throat to readily enter the middle ear, predisposing this age group to more frequent ear infections.

The inner ear contains auditory nerve endings, which pick up sound waves from the middle ear and transmit them along the eighth cranial nerve, or auditory nerve, to the brain. Sound waves that contact the skull directly can also be picked up by the inner ear. The inner ear contains the structures for balance and for hearing.

The three divisions of the ear develop in the embryo at the same time as other vital organs are developing, which is why deformities of the ears can provide clues to developmental aberrations elsewhere in the body. External ear development begins at about the fifth week of gestation, and middle ear development at around the sixth week. The ears are particularly vulnerable to developmental aberration in the ninth week of gestation.

Neonates are capable of sound discrimination at birth and respond more readily to high-pitched voices. The presence of mucus in the eustachian tube may limit hearing when the neonate is first born but clears shortly after birth. Vernix caseosa in the external ear canal may make visualization of the tympanic membrane difficult.

The young infant responds to loud noises with the startle reflex, blinking, or cessation of movement. Infants, 6 months of age or older, attempt to locate the source of the sound.

Equipment for Ear Assessment

Tuning fork
Otoscope
Ear speculum
Bell

Preparation

Ask parents about a family history of hearing problems, maternal infections during pregnancy, problems during labor and delivery, and neonatal jaundice. Ask if the child has had convulsions, unexplained fever, drainage from the ear, mumps, measles, ear and respiratory tract infections, surgery to the ear, and prolonged use of ototoxic drugs.

Inquire as to when the child began speaking and whether there are any current concerns, such as inattentiveness to parental requests.

If an otoscopic examination is to be performed in a young child or infant, it is safer to restrain him or her. Explain and demonstrate to the parent how the child is to be held. The child can be placed on the side or abdomen, with the hands at the side and the head turned so that the ear to be examined points toward

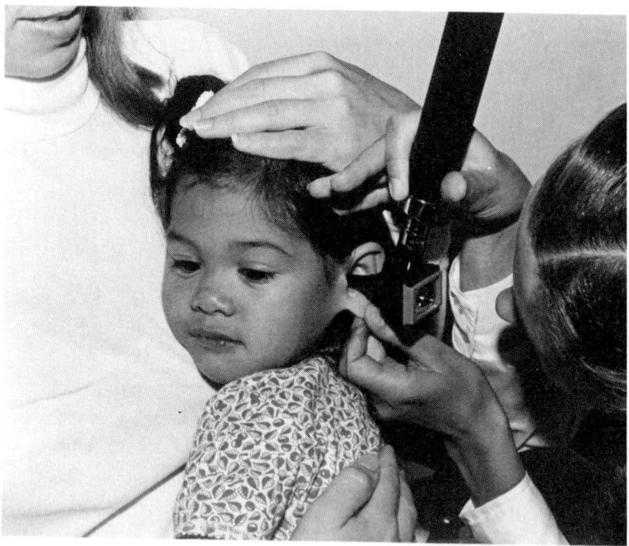

Figure 11-1
Position for restraining infant or child during otoscopic examination.
(From Whaley LF, Wong DL: Nursing care of infants and children, ed 4, St Louis, 1991, Mosby–Year Book.)

the ceiling. The parent can assist by placing one hand on the child's head above the ear and the other on the child's trunk. Alternatively, the child can sit on the parent's lap with one arm tucked behind the parent's back. The parent holds the child's head against his or her shoulder and the child's other, free arm (Figure 11-1).

Assessment of External Ear

Assessment	Findings
Examine the ear for placement and position.	The top of the ear should cross an imaginary line from the inner eye to the occiput. The pinna should deviate no more than 10 degrees from a line perpendicular to the horizontal line. (Use of a pen or tongue blade can provide more concrete estimations of where the ear is positioned in relation to a vertical line.) Figure 11-2 illustrates normal placement and position of the ear. **Clinical Alert** Low or obliquely set ears are sometimes seen in children with genitourinary or chromosomal abnormalities and in many syndromes.
Observe the ears for protrusion or flattening.	The ears of neonates are flat against the head. **Clinical Alert** Flattened ears in older infants may suggest persistent side-lying. Protruding ears may indicate swelling related to insect bites or to conditions such as mastoiditis.

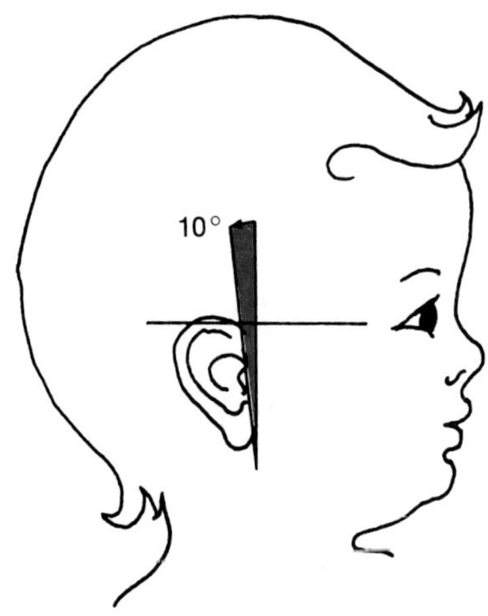

Figure 11-2
Ear placement and position.
(From Whaley LF, Wong DL: Nursing care of infants and children, ed 4, St Louis, 1991, Mosby–Year Book.)

Assessment	Findings
Inspect the external ear for unusual structure and markings. Figure 11-3 illustrates usual markings.	Markings and structure of the external ear vary little from child to child. Variations may be normal but should be recorded. For example, a small skin tag on the tragus is a remnant of embryonic development. Skinfolds may be absent from the helix. Parents and child may be sensitive about this abnormality.
Inspect the external ear canal for general hygiene, discharge, and excoriations.	The skin of the external auditory meatus (Figure 11-3) is normally flesh colored. Soft yellow-brown wax is normal.

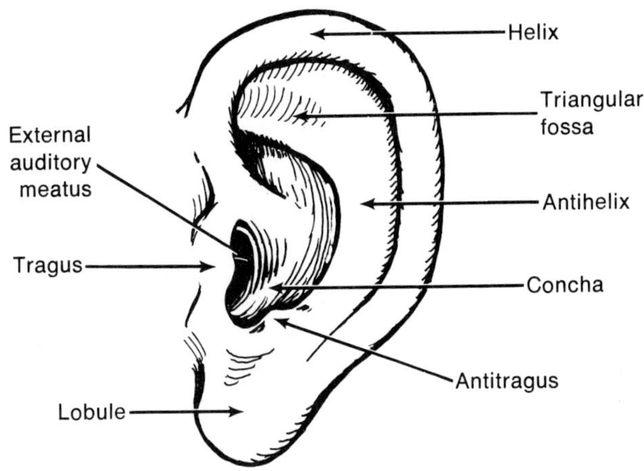

Figure 11-3
Usual landmarks of pinna.
(From Whaley LF, Wong DL: Nursing care of infants and children, ed 4, St Louis, 1991, Mosby–Year Book.)

Assessment	Findings
	Clinical Alert Absence of wax in the external ear may indicate overly vigorous cleaning. Hygienic measures can best be determined by commenting on how clean the ears are and then asking how the ears are cleaned. Parents may need teaching about the dangers of using sharp objects. Advise use of a soft washcloth. Absence of wax may also be related to acute otitis media. If cleaning practices are acceptable, ask about ear pulling, irritability, and fever.

Assessment	Findings
	Foul-smelling yellow or green discharge may indicate rupture of a tympanic membrane or recent insertion of myringotomy tubes.
	Bloody discharge may indicate foreign body irritation or scratching.
Pull on the auricle	Pulling normally produces no pain.
	Clinical Alert Pain produced by pulling on the auricle may indicate otitis externa.
Palpate the bony protruberance behind the ear (mastoid) for tenderness.	No pain or tenderness should be experienced when the mastoid is palpated.
	Clinical Alert Pain and tenderness over the mastoid process may indicate mastoiditis.

Assessment of Hearing Acuity

Hearing loss, the most common handicap, may be of three types. Conduction hearing loss results from disruption of sound transmission through outer and middle ear, most often as the result of serous otitis media. Sensorineural loss is a result of damage to the inner ear or auditory nerve. Mixed loss reflects both conduction and sensorineural hearing loss.

Assessment	Findings
Infant	
Stand behind the child and ring a small bell, snap fingers, or clap hands. Be careful not to bump the examining table,	The infant younger than 4 months evidences a startle reflex. Infants, 6 months of age or older, try to locate the

Assessment	Findings
because this evokes a false response from the infant.	sound by shifting their eyes or turning their heads. The infant may also cease movement in response to sound.
	Clinical Alert
	Suspect hearing loss in a young infant who does not startle or cease movement or who has been premature and in intensive care.
	Suspect hearing loss in an older infant who does not attempt to localize sound.
Preschool-Aged Child	
Stand 0.6 to 0.9 m (2 to 3 ft) in front of the child and give commands, such as "Please give me the doll."	
School-Aged Child or Adolescent	
Stand about 0.3 m (1 ft) behind the child. Instruct the child to cover one ear. Ask the child to repeat what is heard while you whisper numbers in random order. Repeat the process with the other ear.	
Rinne's Test (to compare air and bone conduction)	
Strike the tuning fork against your palm, then hold the stem to the child's mastoid process. When the child indicates that the sound is no longer audible, hold the prongs near the external meatus of one ear and ask the	Normally the child can hear the sound of the tuning fork at the external meatus after it is no longer audible at the mastoid process (positive test result), because air conduction is better than bone conduction.

Assessment	Findings
child if the sound can be heard. Repeat the process with the other ear.	Sound should be heard equally well in both ears (positive test result). **Clinical Alert** Interference with conduction of air through the external and middle chambers causes the child to experience sound better through bone conduction.
Weber's Test (to differentiate conduction from sensorineural deafness)	
Strike the tuning fork against the palm and hold the stem in the midline of the child's head. Ask the child where sound is heard best.	**Clinical Alert** With air conduction loss the sound is heard better in the *affected* ear. The sound is heard best in the *unaffected* ear if loss is sensorineural.

Otoscopic Examination

Many children are apprehensive about the otoscopic examination. Apprehension can be lessened by allowing the child to see and handle the otoscope and to turn the light on and off. Reassure that the examination may tickle but does not hurt. Restrain the infant or young child to prevent sudden movement.

Assessment	Findings
Select the largest speculum that fits comfortably into the ear canal. Hold the otoscope in an inverted position.	The ear canal is normally pink, but may be more pigmented in dark-skinned children, and has minute hairs.

Assessment	Findings
Check the canal opening for foreign bodies.	The tympanic membrane is translucent and pearly pink or gray. Slight redness is normal in the newborn infant and may be normal in older infants and children who have been crying.
Straighten the ear canal. In children younger than 3 years, pull the earlobe gently down and out. In children older than 3 years, pull the pinna up and back. Place the speculum in the canal. In children younger than 3 years, direct the speculum upward, and in children older than 3 years, direct it downward and forward. Avoid sudden movement.	**Clinical Alert** Marked erythema of the tympanic membrane may indicate acute otitis media. A dull yellow or gray tympanic membrane may indicate serous otitis media.
Inspect the ear canal for lesions, discharge, and cerumen.	
Inspect the tympanic membrane for landmarks (Figure 11-4) and color.	

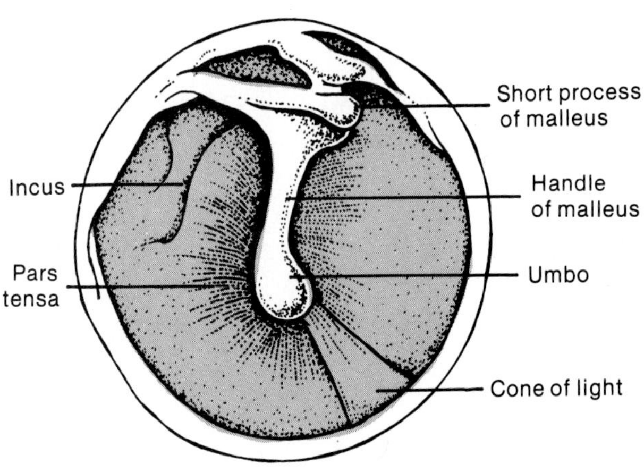

Figure 11-4
Usual landmarks of tympanic membrane.
(From Potter PA: Pocket nurse guide to physical assessment, St Louis, 1990, Mosby–Year Book.)

Related Nursing Diagnoses

Comfort, alteration in: Pain related to infection; pruritis.

Communication, impaired verbal: Related to decreased or absent auditory discrimination; decreased or absent auditory comprehension.

Coping, ineffective family: Related to inability to communicate effectively with child.

Coping, ineffective individual: Related to inability to communicate.

Infection, high risk for: Secondary to contact with contagious agents.

Injury, high risk for: Related to knowledge deficit.

Knowledge deficit: Related to appropriate care of the ear.

Parenting, alteration in: Related to child's inability to communicate; child's inability to hear.

Self-concept, disturbance in self-esteem: Related to perception of physical handicap.

Sensory-perceptual alteration, auditory: Related to alterations in detection of sound.

Skin integrity, impaired: Related to improper cleaning of ear; presence of irritating drainage.

Social interaction, impaired: Related to communication difficulties.

Eyes

12

Assessment of the eye involves examination of the external and internal eye, visual acuity, extraocular movement, position, alignment, and color vision.

Rationale

Disorders of vision can interfere with a child's ability to respond to stimuli and to learn and with the ability to perform activities of daily living independently. Early detection and referral can minimize the effects of deficiencies in vision. Vision disturbances can alert health practitioners to underlying congenital and acquired disorders.

Anatomy and Physiology

The eye is composed of three layers. The first, outermost layer consists of the sclera, or white of the eye, which is opaque, and of the cornea, which is transparent (Figure 12-1). Underlying the cornea is the iris, which is colored and muscular. At its center is the pupil. The lens lies posterior to the pupil, suspended by ciliary muscles. A final layer, the retina, contains rods and cones, which receive visual stimuli and send them to the brain via the optic nerve. The fovea centralis, which appears as a small depression at the back of the retina, contains the greatest number of cones. The macula immediately surrounds the fovea centralis. The optic nerve enters the orb through the optic disk. Six muscles hold the eyes in position in their sockets. Coordinated movement of the muscles produces binocular vision. The eyelid, which protects the eye, is lined with the conjunctiva, which is vascular.

At 22 days of gestation the eye appears, and by 8 weeks as-

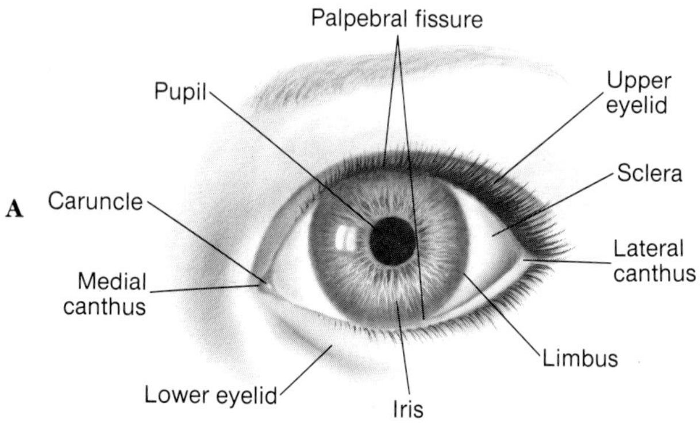

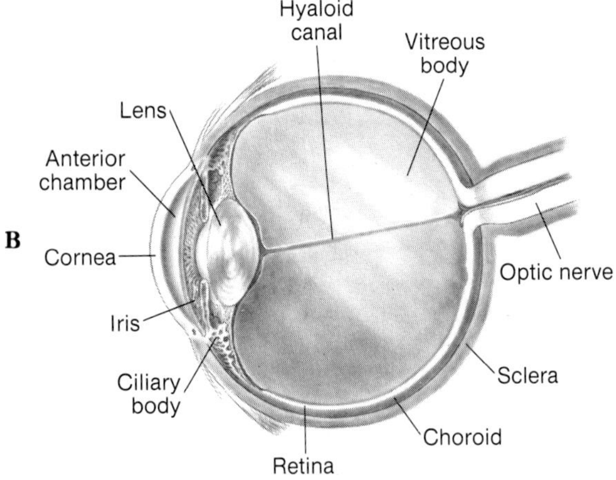

Figure 12-1
Normal structure of eye. A, Anterior view. B, Cross-sectional view.
(From Whaley LF, Wong DL: Nursing care of infants and children, ed 4, St Louis, 1991, Mosby–Year Book.)

sumes its familiar form. Its structure and form continue to evolve until the child reaches school age. At birth myelinization of the nerve fibers is complete and a pupillary response can be elicited. The newborn infant, however, has limited vision. The neonate is

Table 12-1 Visual acuity in infants and children

Age	Visual Acuity
Birth	Infant fixates on objects 0.2 to 0.3 m (8 to 12 in) away (such as mother's face)
4 mo	20/300 to 20/50
2 yr	20/70
4 yr	20/40
5 yr	20/30 to 20/20

able to identify the mother's form and is aware of light and motion, as evidenced by the blink reflex. Searching nystagmus is common. The definitive ability to follow objects is not developed until about 4 weeks of life, when the infant is able to follow light and objects to midline. By 8 weeks the infant is able to follow light past midline, although strabismus may be evident.

Intermittent convergent strabismus is common until 6 months of age, then disappears. The muscles assume completely mature function by 1 year. The macula and fovea centralis are structurally differentiated by 4 months. Macular maturation is achieved by 6 years of age. Color discrimination is present between 3 and 5 months. The infant is normally farsighted. Like small children, infants see well at close range. Visual acuity in infants ranges from 20/300 to 20/50 (Table 12-1). The iris usually assumes permanent color by 6 months, but in some children not until 1 year. Lacrimation is present by 6 to 12 weeks of age.

Equipment for Eye Assessment

Penlight
Visual acuity chart (choice of chart based on age of child)
  Snellen's chart
  Snellen E chart
  Allen cards
Index card
Cotton-tipped applicator
Ophthalmoscope
Ishihara's test (for color vision)

Preparation

Ask the parent or child if the child is clumsy, sits close to the television, has difficulty seeing the board (school-aged child), or responds to approaching objects without blinking (infant). Ask about the presence of pain, discharge, excessive tearing, squinting, blurred or double vision, burning, itching, and light sensitivity. Inquire whether there is a family history of vision problems (glaucoma, color blindness). Alert the physician to any of these symptoms.

Assessment of External Eye

Assessment	Findings
Position and Placement	
Note whether the eyes are wide set (hypertelorism) or close set (hypotelorism). Measure the distance between the inner canthi, if in doubt (Figure 12-2).	Inner canthal distance averages 2.5 cm (1 inch). **Clinical Alert** Hypertelorism is present in Down syndrome.

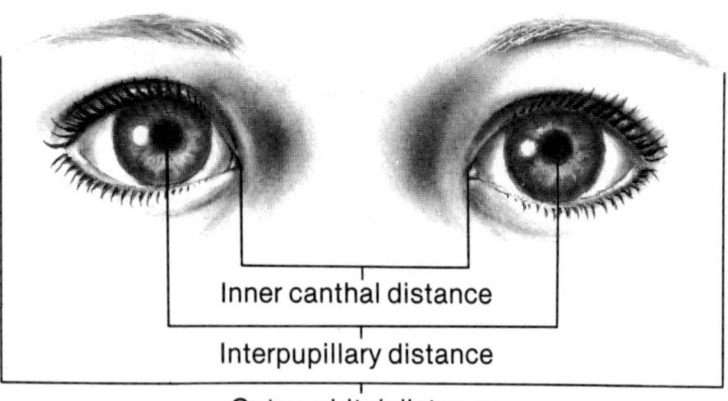

Figure 12-2
Anatomical landmarks of eye.
(From Whaley LF, Wong DL: Nursing care of infants and children, ed 4, St Louis, 1991, Mosby–Year Book.)

Assessment	Findings
Observe for vertical folds that partially or completely cover the inner canthi.	Epicanthal folds are normally seen in Oriental children and in some non-Oriental children. **Clinical Alert** Epicanthal folds may indicate Down syndrome, renal agenesis, or glycogen storage disease.
Observe the slant of the eyes by drawing an imaginary line across the inner canthi (Figure 12-3).	The palpebral fissures lie horizontally along the imaginary line. Oriental children normally have an upward slant to their eyes. **Clinical Alert** Upward slant of the eyes is present in Down syndrome.
Observe the eyelids for proper placement.	The eyelid falls between the upper border of the iris and the upper border of the pupil.

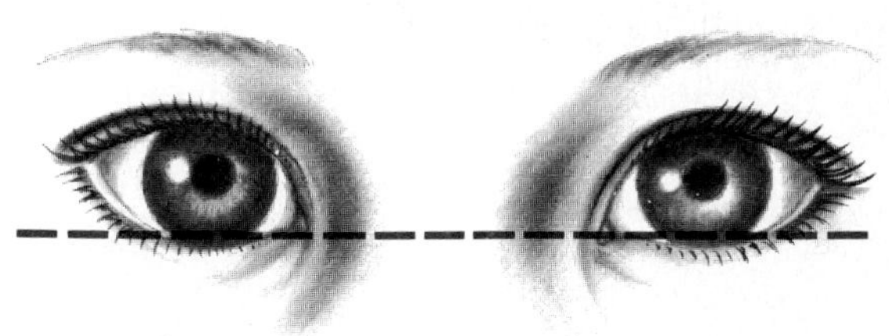

Figure 12-3
Upward palpebral slant.
(From Whaley LF, Wong DL: Nursing care of infants and children, ed 4, St Louis, 1991, Mosby–Year Book.)

Assessment	Findings
	Clinical Alert Appearance of sclera between the upper lid and iris (sunset sign) is present in hydrocephalus, although it may be a normal variant. Drooping of the eyelid over the pupil (ptosis) may be a normal variant or may signal a variety of disorders, such as paralysis of the oculomotor cranial nerve. If the eyelids turn inward (entropion), the corners can become irritated by the eyelashes. If the eyelids turn outward (ectropion), the conjunctiva is exposed.
Eyebrows	
Inspect the eyebrows for symmetry and hair growth.	Eyebrows normally are shaped and move symmetrically. They do not meet in midline.
Eyelids	
Observe distribution and condition of eyelashes.	Eyelashes curl outward.
Inspect eyelids for color, swelling, discharge, and lesions.	Eyelids normally are the same color as the surrounding skin. **Clinical Alert** Flat pink areas on eyelids may be telangiectatic nevi or "stork bite marks," which disappear by 1 year of age. A painful, red, swollen eyelid may indicate a stye. A nodular nontender area may be a chalazion (cyst).

Assessment	Findings
	Swelling, redness, and purulent discharge may be related to inflammation of the lacrimal sac (dacryocystitis), often the result of a blocked tear duct, which may disappear as an infant reaches 6 months of age.
	If the area around the eyelids appears sunken, the child may be dehydrated.
	Shadow under the eyes may indicate fatigue or allergy.
Conjunctivae	
Inspect the lower lid by pulling down as the child looks up. Inspect the upper lid by rolling the eyelid over a cotton-tipped applicator.	The conjunctivae should be pink and glossy.
	Clinical Alert
	Redness of the conjunctivae may be related to bacterial or viral infection, allergy, or irritation.
	A cobblestone appearance of the conjunctivae may accompany severe allergy.
	Excessive pallor of the conjunctivae may accompany anemia.
Inspect the bulbar conjunctivae for color.	The bulbar conjunctivae should be clear and transparent, allowing the white of the sclerae to be clearly visible.
	Clinical Alert
	Redness may indicate fatigue, eyestrain, irritation, or bleeding disorders.
	Overgrowth of conjunctival tissue (pterygium) can cover the cornea.

Assessment	Findings
Inspect the sclerae for color.	The sclerae should be white and clear. Tiny black marks in dark-skinned children are normal. **Clinical Alert** Yellow appearance may indicate jaundice. Bluish discoloration may indicate osteogenesis imperfecta, glaucoma, or later stages of increased bilirubin.
Pupils and Irises	
Inspect the irises for color, shape, and inflammation.	Irises of different colors may be normal. Irises should be round and clear. **Clinical Alert** A notch at the outer edge of the iris (coloboma) may indicate a visual field defect and should be reported. White or light speckling of the iris (Brushfield's spots) may indicate Down syndrome. Absence of color and a pinkish glow may indicate albinism.
Inspect the pupils for size, equality, and response to light. Observe and record the pupil size in normal room light. Darken the room and observe the response of each pupil when light is directly shone into it (direct light reflex) and when light is shone into the opposite eye (consensual light reflex). Place your	Pupils are normally equal in size, although inequality is not uncommon and may be nonpathologic if other findings are normal. Pupils should respond briskly to light. In the consensual reaction the pupil should constrict when light is shone in the contralateral eye.

Assessment	Findings
nondominant hand down the midline of the nose while performing the test for consensual reaction.	**Clinical Alert** Constriction of the pupils (miosis) may occur with iritis and with morphine administration. Dilation of pupils (mydriasis) may be related to emotional factors, acute glaucoma, some drugs, trauma, circulatory arrest, and anesthesia. Fixed unilateral dilation of a pupil may indicate local eye trauma or head injury.

Assessment of Extraocular Movement

Two tests are commonly used to test binocular vision: the corneal light reflex test and the cover test. The eyes are also assessed for nystagmus (rapid, jerky movements of the eye) through field of vision testing.

Assessment	Findings
Corneal Light Reflex Test	
Assess for strabismus by shining a light directly into the eyes from a distance of about 40.5 cm (16 in). Observe the site of the reflection in each pupil.	Normally the light falls symmetrically on each pupil. Intermittent alternating convergent strabismus is normal during the first 6 months of life. **Clinical Alert** Report any malalignment. If malalignment is present, the light falls off center in one eye and neither eye deviates. Infants with a birth weight of less than 1500 gm (3.3 lb) are more prone to muscle imbalance and warrant early, periodic screening.

Assessment	Findings
Cover Test	
Ask the child to look at your nose; then cover one of the child's eyes. Observe whether the uncovered eye moves. Uncover the occluded eye and inspect for movement.	**Clinical Alert** Movement may indicate strabismus. Record the direction of any eye movement. Refer for further testing.
Field of Vision	
Ask the child to follow a finger or shiny object through the six cardinal fields of gaze (Figure 12-4). Children younger than 2 or 3 years of age may not be able to cooperate with this test. Observe the eye movements of the younger child as the examination progresses.	A few beats of nystagmus in the far lateral gaze are normal. **Clinical Alert** Report easily elicited nystagmus.

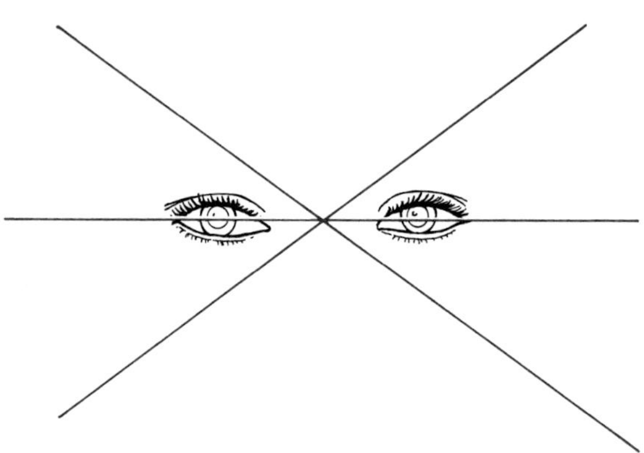

Figure 12-4
Six cardinal fields of gaze.

Assessment of Color Vision

Color vision can be assessed by using Ishihara's test, composed of a set of cards with a series of round dots in the shape of a figure or number. The figures or numbers are not discernible by eyes with impaired color vision.

Assessment of Visual Acuity

Testing of visual acuity in children is not simple and can be directly affected by the child, the nurse, and the environment. There is no simple method to accurately test visual acuity in children younger than 3 years.

Assessment	Findings
Observe whether the infant blinks and exhibits dorsiflexion in response to light.	**Clinical Alert** Report absence of blink reflex.
Observe whether the infant of 4 weeks or older is able to fixate on a brightly colored object and follow it.	**Clinical Alert** Report inability to follow an object and reassess.
Snellen's Test	
Hang the Snellen chart so that it lies smoothly and firmly on a light-colored wall. There should be no glare on the chart. Have the child stand 6.1 m (20 ft) from the chart. Test both eyes first, then the right eye, then the left eye. Unless the child has very poor vision, begin with the line on the chart that corresponds to a distance of 12.2 m (40 ft). The child must be able to see three of four or four of six symbols on a line to correctly visualize the line. Test with glasses or contact lenses if the child wears them.	**Clinical Alert** Refer children with a one-line difference between eyes. Refer 4-year-old children with visual acuity of 20/40 or less.

Assessment	Findings
If using the Snellen E chart, have the child indicate the direction of the E's "legs" with his/her fingers or with a cardboard E. Use the 20/100 E to determine whether the child understands what to do. Proceed as for regular Snellen testing.	
Allen Cards	
Show the child the cards at close range and have the child name the pictures from a distance of 4.6 m (15 ft). Test each eye, if possible.	The child should be able to name three of seven cards in a maximum of five tries.

Ophthalmoscopic Examination

Ophthalmoscopic examination requires practice and patience and a cooperative child. In younger infants and children it may be possible to elicit only the red reflex. The retina, choroid, optic nerve disk, macula, fovea centralis, and retinal vessels are visualized with the ophthalmoscope.

Darken the room. Sit the child on the parent's lap or examination table or lie the child on the table. Use your right hand and eye to examine the child's right eye and your left hand and eye for the left eye. Ask the child to gaze straight ahead.

Assessment	Findings
Set the dial of the ophthalmoscope at 0. Approach from a distance of 30.5 cm (12 in), centering the light in the eye. The pupil glows red (red reflex). Gradually move closer and change the dial of the ophthalmoscope to plus or minus diopters to focus.	In infants the optic disk is pale and the peripheral vessels not well developed. The red reflex appears lighter in infants. In children the red reflex appears as a brilliant, uniform glow. The optic disk is creamy white to pinkish, with clear margins. At the center of the optic disk is a small

Assessment	Findings
	depression (the physiologic cup). Arteries are smaller and brighter than veins. The macula is the same size as the optic disk and to the right of the disk. The fovea is a glistening spot in the center of the macula. **Clinical Alert** Report a partial or white reflex, blurring of the disk margins, bulging of the disk, and hemorrhage. Blockage of the red reflex may be indicative of cataract.

Related Nursing Diagnoses

Comfort, alteration in: Pain, secondary to infection; irritation; trauma.

Coping, ineffective individual: Related to temporary or permanent loss of vision.

Diversional activity deficit: Related to inability to perform usual activities of daily living.

Family processes, alteration in: Related to disabilities caused by loss of vision.

Growth and development, altered: Related to decreased stimulation secondary to loss of vision.

Infection, high risk for: Related to contact with contagious elements; loss of integrity of eye tissue.

Injury, high risk for: Related to inability to see environmental hazards.

Self-care deficit: Related to inability to procure materials needed for self-care; inability to control environment.

Self-concept, disturbance in: Related to loss of vision.

Sensory-perceptual alteration, visual: Secondary to trauma; infection; congenital or acquired disorders of vision.

Social isolation: Related to disturbance in self-concept; inability to control environment.

Face, Nose, and Oral Cavity

13

Rationale

The face provides a map of the child's emotional status and clues to neurologic, congenital, and allergic conditions. The nose provides entry to the respiratory tract, and the mouth provides entry to the digestive tract. Examination of the nose, mouth, and sinuses provides information about the functioning of the respiratory and digestive tracts and about the overall health of the child.

The common occurrence of tonsillitis provides reason enough for inspection of the oropharynx. However, examination of the nose, oral cavity, and oropharynx also yields valuable information about congenital anomalies, nutritional status, hygienic practices, and overall health. The information obtained can be used in the prevention, early detection, and nursing management of such disorders.

Anatomy and Physiology

The face of the newborn infant and child is noticeably different from that of the adult. Typically the neonate appears to have a slightly receding chin. By 6 years of age the mandible and maxilla have grown significantly in length and width and the chin shows greater development. A six-year-old child has approximately 80% of the facial dimensions of the adult.

Sinuses are air pockets adjacent to the nasal passage. Only the ethmoid and maxillary sinuses are present at birth (Figure 13-1). The frontal sinus develops at around 7 years of age, and the sphenoid sinus in adolescence. Development of the sinuses is assisted by enlarging skull bones.

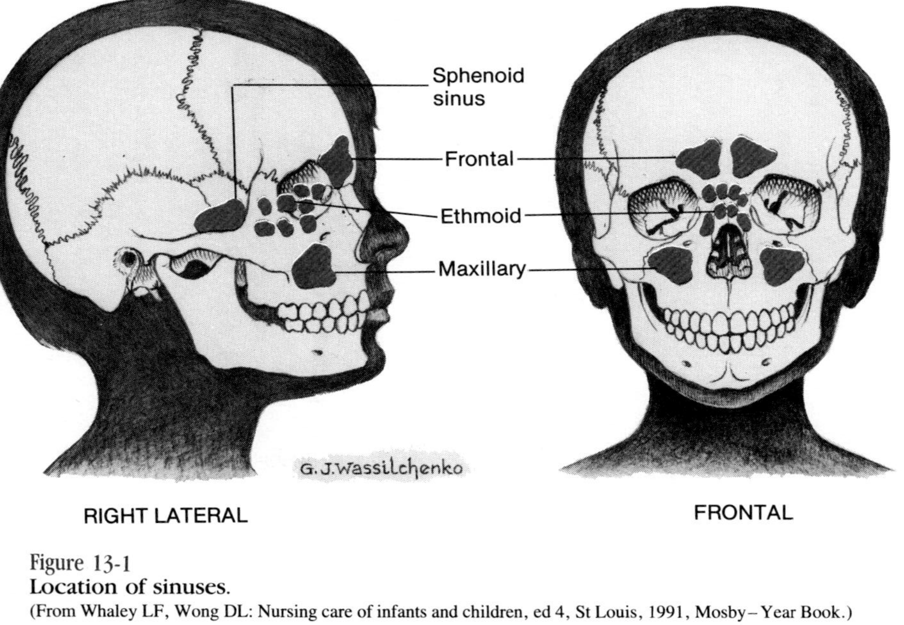

Figure 13-1
Location of sinuses.
(From Whaley LF, Wong DL: Nursing care of infants and children, ed 4, St Louis, 1991, Mosby–Year Book.)

The nose warms, filters, and moistens air entering the respiratory tract and is the organ of smell. Infants have a narrow bridge and are obligate nose breathers, which readily predisposes them to compromise of the upper airway. The sense of smell is poor at birth but develops with age.

The mouth of the young infant is short, smooth, and has a relatively long soft palate. The tongue appears large in the shorter oral cavity and tends to press into the concavity of the roof of the mouth, which allows milk to flow back to the pharynx. By 6 months the mouth is proportioned like that of the adult. Until approximately 4 months of age the infant demonstrates an active tongue thrust, or extrusion reflex, in which the tongue is pressed under the nipple. This reflex is of concern to some parents, who think that the infant is rejecting solid foods by thrusting them out as soon as they are placed on the tongue. By approximately 6 months of age the rhythmic up-and-down sucking motions of the tongue become the more adult forward-backward tongue movement. The rooting reflex, in which the infant turns the mouth in the direction that the cheek is touched, assists in food attainment and is seen in the infant younger than 3 or 4 months.

Typically the infant of 3 months begins to drool as salivation increases. The increased saliva production, together with an inappropriate swallowing reflex and lack of lower teeth, allows saliva to flow outward.

The sense of taste is immature at birth but becomes acute by 2 to 3 months as taste buds mature. However, the sense of taste is not fully functional until approximately 2 years of age, as evidenced by the strange things that young children ingest.

In newborn infants the gingivae (gums) are smooth, with a raised fringe of tissue along the gum line. Pearllike areas may be seen along the gingivae. These are often mistaken for teeth, but are retention cysts and disappear in 1 to 2 months. True dentition begins at approximately 6 months of age, when the lower central incisors appear. By 30 months the child has 20 teeth and primary dentition is complete (Figure 13-2). During middle childhood the permanent molars erupt and the primary teeth are lost. The typical 6-year-old appears toothless. Tooth eruptions and losses are genetically predetermined.

Tonsils are found in the pharyngeal cavity and are part of the lymphatic system. Several pairs make up Waldeyer's tonsillar ring, which encircles the pharynx; but only the palatine, or faucial, tonsil is readily visible behind the faucial pillars in the oropharynx (Figure 13-3). The pharyngeal tonsils and adenoids are located on the posterior wall of the oropharynx. Although tonsillar tissue begins to shrink by approximately 7 years of age, the child normally has larger tonsils and adenoids than either the infant or the adolescent.

Equipment for Face, Nose, and Oral Cavity Assessment

Tongue blade
Penlight
Glove

A

	Age of eruption (mo)	Average age of shedding (yr)
Maxilla	9.6	7.5
	12.4	8
	18.3	11.5
	15.7	10.5
	26.2	10.5
Mandible	26.0	11
	15.1	10
	18.2	9.5
	11.5	7
	7.8	6

Figure 13-2
Primary and secondary dentition. A, Sequence of eruption and shedding of teeth.
(From Whaley LF, Wong DL: Essentials of pediatric nursing, ed 3, St Louis, 1989, Mosby–Year Book.)

Continued.

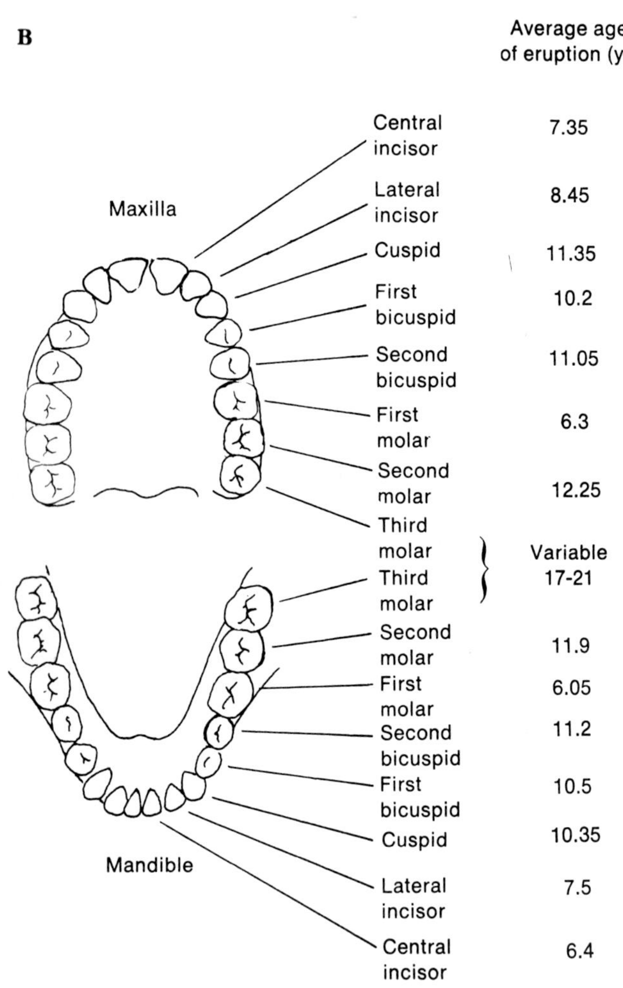

Figure 13-2, cont'd
B, Sequence of eruption of secondary teeth.

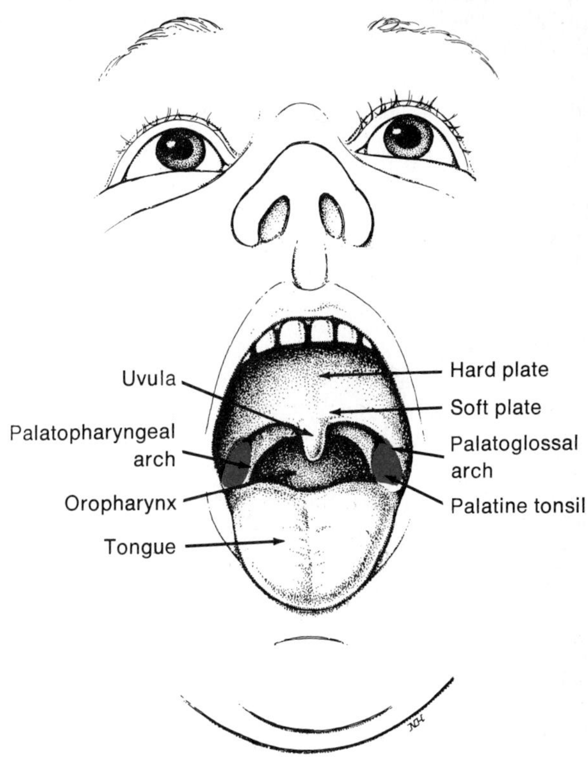

Figure 13-3
Interior structures of mouth.
(From Whaley LF, Wong DL: Nursing care of infants and children, ed 4, St Louis, 1991, Mosby–Year Book.)

Preparation

Inquire whether the child has or has had frequent sore throats, epistaxis, allergies, hay fever, recent contacts with persons with communicable disease, fever, or difficulty in swallowing. Ask about oral hygiene practices and date of last dental visit (if 3 years or older). Ask if the child is receiving medications.

Infants and children find examination of the mouth intrusive, and it is best left until the end of the examination. The nurse often has an opportunity to visualize the oral cavity without a tongue blade when the infant or child cries, laughs, or yawns. Infants and young children are frequently more comfortable on the parent's lap during this part of the examination and can be reclined slightly for a better view. Infants and young children may need restraining.

Assessment of Face and Nose

Assessment	Findings
Observe the spacing and size of facial features.	Infants who were premature may have a narrow forehead. **Clinical Alert** Coarse features combined with a low hairline and large tongue may indicate cretinism. An enlarged forehead may be indicative of hydrocephalus.
Carefully observe the facial expression, especially around the eyes and mouth.	**Clinical Alert** A child with a persistently sad and forlorn expression may be abused, particularly if bruises can be detected on the body. A child who demonstrates an open mouth and facial contortions may be suffering from allergic rhinitis. Shadow under the eyes may indicate fatigue or allergy.
Observe the symmetry of the nasolabial folds as the child cries and smiles.	Normal nasolabial folds are symmetric. **Clinical Alert** Asymmetry of the nasolabial folds may indicate facial nerve impairment or Bell's palsy.

Assessment	Findings
Observe the size and shape of the nose. Draw an imaginary line down the center of the face between the eyes and down the notch of the upper lip.	The nose should be symmetric and in the center of the face. A flattened bridge is sometimes seen in Oriental and black children. **Clinical Alert** A flattened nose may indicate congenital anomalies and should be reported.
Observe the external nares for flaring, discharge, excoriation, and odor.	**Clinical Alert** Flaring external nares indicate respiratory distress. The skin of the external nares should be intact. No discharge should be seen, although a clear, watery discharge may be present if the child has been crying. Excoriation of the external nares may indicate the presence of an irritating discharge and frequent nose wiping. A clear, thin, nasal discharge is often present with allergic rhinitis. Purulent yellow or green discharge accompanies infection. Clear nasal discharge following a head injury may be cerebrospinal fluid. A foul odor may indicate the presence of a foreign body.
Test the patency of the nares by placing the diaphragm of the stethoscope under one nostril while blocking the other. A film appears on the diaphragm if the naris is patent.	Both nares should be patent.

Assessment	Findings
Tilt the head backward and push the tip of the nose upward to visualize the internal nasal cavity. Use a penlight for better illumination. Observe the integrity, color, and consistency of the mucosa and the position of the septum.	The nasal mucosa should be firm and pink. **Clinical Alert** A pale, boggy nasal mucosa indicates allergic rhinitis. A red mucosa indicates infection. Excoriation of the nasal mucosa may indicate nose picking, a common cause of epistaxis in children. Grayish soft outgrowths of mucosa are polyps that may partially obstruct the nares. Report any deviation of the nasal septum.
Ask older children about their sense of smell. Test the sense of smell by having the child close eyes. Block one nostril at a time and ask the child to identify distinctive odors such as coffee and lemon. The child should be able to correctly identify each.	**Clinical Alert** Diminished smell may indicate olfactory nerve impairment.
Palpate above the eyebrows and each side of the nose to determine if pain and tenderness are present.	**Clinical Alert** Pain and tenderness in these regions may indicate sinusitis.

Related Nursing Diagnoses

Airway clearance, ineffective: Related to decreased nasal patency; swollen mucous membranes.

Anxiety: Related to air hunger.

Infection, high risk for: Related to contact with contagious agents.

Sensory-perceptual alteration, olfactory: Secondary to olfactory nerve impairment; obstruction; sinusitis.

Skin integrity, impaired: Related to irritating nasal secretions.

Assessment of Oral Cavity

Assessment	Findings
Inspect the lips for color, symmetry, moisture, swelling, sores, and fissures.	The lips should be intact, pink, and firm. **Clinical Alert** Blueness of the lips is a reliable sign of cyanosis in white children. Pallor may indicate anemia. Cherry red coloration is seen with acidosis. Cracked lips are usually the result of harsh climate, lip biting, mouth breathing, or fever. Fissures at the corners of the mouth may indicate deficiency of riboflavin or niacin. Drooping of one side of the lips indicates facial nerve impairment.
Inspect the buccal margins, gingivae, tongue, and palate for moisture, color, intactness, and bleeding. Use a glove and penlight for clearer visualization of any suspected abnormalities. Observe for the presence of odor or halitosis.	The oral membranes are normally pink, firm, smooth, and moist. **Clinical Alert** White ulcerated sores on the oral mucosa are cankers, related to mild trauma, viral infection, or local irritants. Small grayish areas rimmed with red and found on the inner cheek opposite the second molar are Koplik's spots and are indicative of the onset of measles.

Assessment	Findings
	White curdy patches on the gum margins, inner cheeks, tongue, or palate usually indicate thrush (oral moniliasis). Thrush is common in infants (particularly during or following antibiotic therapy), but in children could indicate a deficient immune system disorder such as acquired immune deficiency syndrome (AIDS) or infection with human immunodeficiency virus (HIV). These patches may be distinguished from milk curds in that they cannot be easily scraped away.
	Swelling of gum tissue may be related to anticonvulsant therapy.
	Reddened, swollen, bleeding gums may indicate infection, poor nutrition, or poor oral hygiene.
	A red tongue is related to vitamin deficiencies and to scarlet fever ("strawberry tongue").
	A gray, furrowed, tongue may be normal or may indicate drug ingestion, allergy, or fever.
	Clefts or notches in the hard or soft palate should be noted. An abnormally high, narrow arch may cause problems with sucking in the infant and with speech in the older child.

Assessment	Findings
	Odor or halitosis can indicate poor oral hygiene, constipation, dehydration, sinusitis, food trapped in tonsillar crypts, or systemic illness.
	Drooling accompanied by fever and respiratory distress is indicative of epiglottitis.
Inspect the tongue for movement and size. The older child can be asked to reach the tip of the tongue to the roof of mouth.	The frenulum attaches to the undersurface of the tongue or near its tip, allowing the child to reach the areolar ridge with the tip of the tongue.
Observe the movement of the tongue in infants and younger children as they vocalize or cry.	**Clinical Alert** Inability to touch the tongue to the areolar ridge may signify tongue tie and later speech problems.
	Glossoptosis, or tongue protrusion, is seen in mental retardation and cerebral palsy.
Inspect the teeth for number, type, condition, and occlusion. To estimate the number of teeth that should be present in a child 2 years of age or younger, subtract 6 months from the child's age in months. Ask the child who is 5 years or older if teeth are loose. To assess malocclusion, ask the child to bite down hard.	A normal 30-month-old child has 20 temporary teeth. A child with full permanent dentition has 32 teeth. The upper teeth should slightly override the lower teeth.
	Clinical Alert Brown and black spots usually indicate caries. Mottling may indicate excessive fluoride intake. Green and black staining can accompany oral iron intake.

Assessment	Findings
	Protrusion of the lower teeth or marked protrusion of the upper teeth should be noted.
Tonsils may be inspected in the older child by asking the child to say "ahh." If the child has difficulty holding the tongue down, the tongue can be *lightly* depressed with the tongue blade on either side. Playing games and demonstrating what is expected of the child through the use of a parent or doll can be very useful. If the nurse is unable to observe the tonsil bed while the infant or older child is crying, the tongue blade can be slid between the lips, along the side of the gum to the back of the mouth, and then quickly slipped between the gums. This produces a gag reflex, which allows the nurse to see the tonsils very well. *Any inspection of the pharynx that involves use of the tongue blade and that may elicit the gag reflex must not be performed in a child who is suspected to have any of the croup syndromes.* Producing the gag reflex in a child with epiglottitis could produce total laryngeal obstruction.	Tonsils, if present, are normally the same color as the buccal mucosa. They are large in the preschool- and school-aged child and appear larger as they move toward the uvula. Crypts may be present on their surface. **Clinical Alert** Reddened tonsils covered with exudate indicate infection. Thick, gray, exudate may indicate diphtheric tonsillitis. Visualization of adenoids suggests that they are enlarged. If adenoids are visualized during gagging or saying "ahh," they appear as grape-like structures.

Assessment	Findings
Observe movement of the uvula during examination of the tonsils.	The uvula remains in midline. **Clinical Alert** Deviation of the uvula or absence of movement may signal involvement of the glossopharyngeal or vagus nerves.
Observe the quality of the voice.	**Clinical Alert** A nasal quality to the voice suggests enlarged adenoids. A hoarse cry or voice may indicate croup, cretinism, or tetany. A shrill, high-pitched cry may indicate increased intracranial pressure.

Related Nursing Diagnoses

Airway clearance, ineffective: Related to swelling.

Comfort, alteration in: Pain related to infection; inflammation.

Communication, impaired verbal: Related to pain; anxiety; tongue tie.

Coping, ineffective family: Related to situational crisis.

Fluid volume deficit: Related to reluctance to drink; inability to swallow secondary to pain and swelling.

Infection: Related to contact with contagious agents.

Knowledge deficit: Related to oral hygiene; alleviation of symptoms of respiratory distress.

Nutrition, alterations in: Less than body requirements related to increased metabolic needs; reluctance or inability to swallow; loss of tissue integrity.

Oral mucous membranes, alteration in: Related to infection; fever; dehydration.

Sensory-perceptual alteration, gustatory and olfactory: Related to infection; diminished taste.

Swallowing, impaired: Related to pain; swelling; neuromuscular dysfunction.

Thorax and Lungs

14

Assessment of the respiratory system includes close observation of the child's behavior and assessment of the thorax and the anterior and posterior chest.

Rationale

Respiratory disorders are common in infancy and in childhood and can be acute, life threatening, or chronic. Early screening and detection are essential to being able to refer children for medical treatment. Knowledgeable assessment also assists in monitoring the progress of treatment.

Anatomy and Physiology

Lungs have two main functions: to supply the body with oxygen and eliminate carbon dioxide and to maintain the body's acid-base balance. The lungs are paired and symmetric. The right lung has three lobes, and the left lung two lobes. Air enters the lungs via the trachea and larynx from the mouth or nose. The trachea gives rise to two major bronchi. The right bronchus is shorter, wider, and angled less sharply to the side than the left.

Fetal lung buds first arise in the fourth week of gestation. Subsequent budding and branching give rise to the mainstem bronchi pulmonary lobules. Branching continues into early childhood, although it is less proliferative. From the sixth month on, the lobules have developed aveolar ducts, and the ducts have developed alveolar sacs, which become true alveoli in the second month of postnatal life.

As the alveolar sacs develop, the epithelium lining the sacs thins. Pulmonary capillaries press into the walls of the sacs as the lungs are prepared for the exchange of oxygen and carbon dioxide, near the end of the sixth month of gestation. During the final weeks of gestation the lungs secrete surfactants that prevent the alveolar sacs from collapsing during expiration, causing atelectasis among other disorders. At birth the lungs are fluid filled. This fluid is rapidly dispelled and absorbed as the lungs fill with air.

The newborn infant's thoracic cage is nearly round. Gradually the transverse diameter increases until the chest assumes the elliptic shape of the adult, at about 6 years of age. The infant's thoracic cage is also relatively soft, which allows it to pull in during labored breathing. Infants have relatively less tissue and cartilage in the trachea and bronchi, which allow these structures to collapse more readily.

Airways tend to grow faster than the vertebral column. In infancy the bifurcation of the trachea is at the level of the third thoracic vertebra. By adulthood the bifurcation is at the level of the fourth thoracic vertebra.

Infants are obligatory nose breathers, and their nasal passages are narrower. Breathing is less rhythmic than in the child. In infants and children under the age of 6 or 7 years, respirations are chiefly diaphragmatic or abdominal. The volume of oxygen expired by the infant and the child is greater than that expired by the adult. The volume of air that is inspired increases as the child grows. At the age of 12 years the child has approximately nine times the number of alveoli that were present at birth.

Equipment for Assessment of Thorax and Lungs

Stethoscope

Preparation

Ask the parent or child about cough, fever, shortness of breath, difficulty in breathing, wheezing, easy fatigability, past respiratory tract infections, frequent colds, and family history of respiratory disorders.

Allow the younger child to play with the stethoscope before performing the assessment. Children often enjoy listening to the sounds in their chests and in their parents' or the nurse's chest. Remove the child's shirt or blouse for best visualization of the chest. Infants and toddlers are often best assessed while held by their parents.

Assessment of Thorax and Lungs

Assessment	Findings
Assess the chest for stridor (high-pitched crowing sound), grunting hoarseness, snoring, wheezing, and cough. Precisely describe the sounds and their occurrence.	**Clinical Alert** Stridor, hoarseness, and a barking cough accompany croup. Inspiratory stridor and expiratory snoring are indicative of epiglottitis. Wheezing may indicate asthma, bronchiolitis, or foreign body aspiration.
Observe the external nares for flaring.	**Clinical Alert** Flaring indicates respiratory distress.
Observe the nailbeds for color and for clubbing (widening and lengthening) of the terminal phalanges (Figure 14-1).	**Clinical Alert** Cyanosis (bluish coloration of nailbeds) is sometimes indicative of respiratory failure. Cyanosis may also be related to vasoconstriction or polycythemia. Clubbing is usually indicative of chronic hypoxemia, as in cystic fibrosis and bronchiectasis.

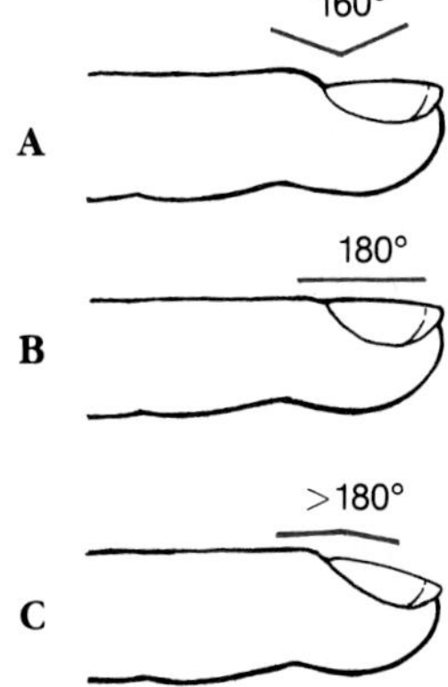

Figure 14-1
Clubbing of nails. **A,** Normal nail. Angle between nail and nail base is approximately 160 degrees. **B,** Early clubbing. Angle between nail and nail base is almost 180 degrees, caused by tissue proliferation on terminal phalanx. **C,** Late clubbing. Angle between nail and nail base is less than 180 degrees. Nail base is visibly swollen.

Assessment	Findings
Observe the color of the child's trunk.	**Clinical Alert** Mottling and cyanosis of the trunk are indicative of severe hypoxemia.
Inspect the thorax for configuration, symmetry, and abnormalities.	The chest is rounder in young children. By 6 years of age the ratio of anteroposterior diameter to transverse diameter is about 1:1.36. In some infants the sternum may be so pliant that the chest appears to cave in with each breath. The thorax should move symmetrically. **Clinical Alert** A round chest in an older child is usually indicative of a chronic lung disorder. A protruberant sternum (pectus carinatum, or pigeon breast) or depressed sternum (pectus excavatum) should be noted. Either may compromise lung expansion. Decreased movement of one side of the thorax may indicate pneumonia, pneumothorax, or a foreign body.
Note the size of the breasts in relation to the age of the child.	Enlarged breasts may be seen in the young infant as a result of maternal hormonal influences. **Clinical Alert** Enlarged breasts (gynecomastia) in older male children may be indicative of obesity or of hormonal or systemic problems.

Assessment	Findings
Observe the chest for retractions, or indrawings, in the supraclavicular (above the clavicles), tracheal (in the sternal notch), substernal (below the sternum), and intercostal (between the ribs) areas (Figure 14-2). Puffiness or bulging of these areas may also be present.	**Clinical Alert** Retractions are an indication of labored breathing in infants and children. Puffiness accompanies severe air trapping.
Observe the child for type of breathing.	In children younger than 7 years respirations are diaphragmatic and the abdomen rises with inspiration. In girls older than 7 years breathing becomes

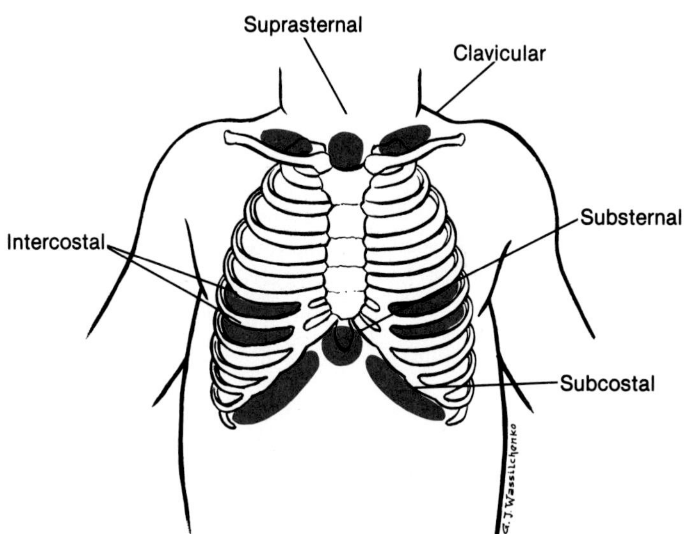

Figure 14-2
Areas where retractions are found.
(From Whaley LF, Wong DL: Nursing care of infants and children, ed 4, St Louis, 1991, Mosby–Year Book.)

Assessment	Findings
	thoracic. Abdomen and chest should move together regardless of type of breathing. **Clinical Alert** Abdominal breathing in an older child may indicate a respiratory disorder or fractured rib. In labored abdominal breathing the abdomen pushes out abruptly.
Observe the depth and regularity of respirations and the duration of inspiration in relation to expiration.	**Clinical Alert** A prolonged expiratory phase may indicate an obstructive respiratory problem, such as asthma.
Palpation	
To assess respiratory excursion, place your hands, thumbs together, along the costal margins of the child's chest or back while the child is sitting.	Movement is symmetric with each breath. Posterior base descends approximately 6 cm (2.3 in) during deep inspiration.
Palpate for tactile fremitus by using either the fingertips or the palmar surfaces of your hands. Move symmetrically while the child says "99" or "blue moon." In the infant, fremitus may be felt as the infant cries.	Fremitus is normally less at the base of the lung. **Clinical Alert** Decreased fremitus may indicate asthma, pneumothorax, or a foreign body. Increased fremitus occurs with pneumonia and atelectasis.
Percussion	
Percussion is more useful in older children. Using the indirect method, percuss the anterior and posterior chest.	Resonance (a low, long sound) is heard over all lung surfaces. Dullness may be heard over the fifth right intercostal space,

Assessment	Findings
Percuss over the intercostal spaces, moving symmetrically and systematically. The child may sit or lie while the anterior chest is percussed, and sit while the posterior chest is percussed.	because of the liver, and over the second to fifth left intercostal space, because of the heart. Tympany (a loud, musical sound) may be heard over the sixth left intercostal space. **Clinical Alert** The percussion note is dull if fluid or a mass is present in the lungs.
Auscultation	
Using the diaphragm of the stethoscope, auscultate the lung fields systematically and *symmetrically* from apex to base. Children can be encouraged to breathe deeply by pretending to blow up balloons or blow out candles.	Breath sounds (Table 14-1) normally seem louder and harsher in the infant and young child, because of the thinness of the chest wall. **Clinical Alert** Report any adventitious sounds (Table 14-2 on pp. 146-147) or breath sounds heard in other than expected areas. If unable to name the sound heard, describe it. Asymmetric rhonchi or wheezes may signal presence of a foreign body.
Auscultate the axillae of children with pneumonia. Rales or crackles may be easily heard in these areas.	
Sounds may be referred from the upper respiratory tract if a child has mucus in the nose or throat. To determine if sounds are referred, place the diaphragm near the child's mouth. Referred sounds are loudest near their origin.	Unilaterally absent breath sounds may indicate pneumothorax.

Table 14-1 Breath sounds

Sound	Relationship of Inspiration to Expiration	Diagram of Sound	Location	
			Normal	Abnormal
Vesicular	Inspiration > Expiration	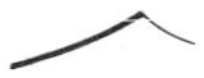	Throughout lung field	None
Bronchovesicular	Inspiration = Expiration	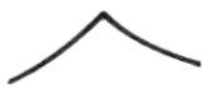	First or second intercostal space, at level of bifurcation of trachea	Peripheral lung
Bronchotubular	Inspiration < Expiration	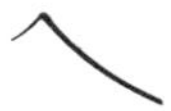	Over trachea	Lung area

Related Nursing Diagnoses

Activity intolerance: Related to breathlessness; fatigue secondary to respiratory infection or obstruction.

Airway clearance, ineffective: Related to secretions; physical alterations of the chest wall; limited expansion of the chest wall.

Anxiety: Related to breathlessness.

Body temperature, high risk for alteration in: Related to infection; inflammation.

Fear: Related to loss of control.

Gas exchange, impaired: Related to exudate; swelling; obstruction.

Growth and development, alteration in: Impaired related to chronic lack of oxygen.

Home maintenance program, altered: Related to home oxygen therapy; medication administration.

Infection, high risk: Related to contact with contagious agents.

Knowledge deficit: Related to therapies; medication; recognition of symptoms.

Parenting, alteration in: Related to situational crisis.

Tissue perfusion, alteration in: Cardiopulmonary related to swelling and exudate secondary to infection and inflammation.

Table 14-2 Adventitious sounds

Sound	Characteristics	Cause
Rales (crackles)		
Fine	Intermittent, high-pitched, soft popping sounds. Heard late in inspiration. Indicative of fluid in alveoli.	Pneumonia, congestive heart failure
Medium	Intermittent, wet, loud, noncrackling, medium pitched. Heard in early or mid-inspiration. Clear with coughing. Indicative of fluid in bronchioles and bronchi.	Pulmonary edema
Coarse	Loud, bubbling, low pitched. Heard on expiration. Clear with coughing. Indicative of fluid in bronchioles and bronchi.	Resolving pneumonia, bronchitis

Rhonchi (wheezes)		
Sonorous	Continuous, snoring, low pitched. Heard throughout respiratory cycle. Clear with coughing. Indicative of involvement of large bronchi and trachea. May also be normal.	Bronchitis
Sibilant	Continuous, musical, high pitched. Heard in mid- to late expiration. Indicative of edema and obstruction in smaller airways. May be audible without a stethoscope.	Asthma
Audible wheezes		
Inspiratory	Sonorous, musical. Heard on inspiration.	High obstruction
Expiratory	Whistling, sighing. Heard during expiration.	Low obstruction
Pleural friction rub	Grating, rubbing, loud, high pitched. May be heard during both inspiration and expiration.	Inflamed pleural surfaces

Table [illegible] Heart sounds

Sound	Cause	Location	Characteristic
S_1 (lubb)	Mitral and tricuspid valves are forced closed at the beginning of systole (contraction).	Apex of heart.	S_1 is longer and lower pitched than S_2. Synchronous with carotid pulse. Closure of valves usually heard as one sound, but slight asynchrony may produce audible splitting, best heard in the fourth left interspace.
S_2 (dubb)	Aortic and pulmonic valves are forced closed at the beginning of diastole (heart relaxation).	Base of heart.	Short, high-pitched S_2 may be split during inspiration. Splitting is best heard in the aortic area. If the breath is held on inspiration, "physiologic split" is accentuated.
S_3	Vibrations are produced by rapid ventricular filling.	Apex of heart.	Heard early in diastole. Dull, low-pitched. Normal in children and young adults.
S_4	Resistance to ventricular filling after contraction of atria.	Apex of heart.	Low pitched. Considered abnormal. Best heard when child is supine.

Cardiovascular System

15

The heart is the primary focus of cardiovascular assessment in the infant and child. Assessment of peripheral circulation may be necessitated under conditions such as application of casts. Auscultation provides the most significant data on cardiac status and receives the most emphasis, yet the importance of other assessments cannot be overlooked.

Rationale

It is estimated that 50% of all children have innocent heart murmurs. Screening and referral of children with murmurs assists in distinguishing between innocent and organic murmurs. Assessment of cardiac and vascular function is an essential component of many hospitalizations, particularly when surgery is performed and when drugs are administered. When cardiac problems have been identified, knowledgeable assessment aids in monitoring the effectiveness of treatment regimens and in early detection of complications.

Anatomy and Physiology

The heart is a muscular four-chambered organ located in the mediastinum. The upper chambers of the heart are the atria, and the lower chambers are the ventricles. Septa divide the two ventricles and the two atria. Four valves prevent the backflow of blood into the chambers. The tricuspid valve, located between the right atrium and ventricle, and the bicuspid, or mitral valve, located between the left atrium and ventricle, are the atrioventricular valves. The pulmonic valve, located in the pulmonary artery, and the aortic valve, in the aorta, are the semilunar valves. Closure of the four valves produces vibrations that are thought to be respon-

sible for heart sounds. S_1 refers to the "lubb"
closure of the atrioventricular valves, and S_2 t
produced by closure of the semilunar valves.
rizes the various sounds and their characterist

In its initial stage of development the hea
Between the second and tenth weeks of gest
series of changes to become a four-chamber
begins beating during the third week of ges
life it primarily distributes the oxygen and
been supplied through the placenta. The fe
bypassed by shunts that exist during fetal
shunts begin to close as pulmonary vascu
Pulmonary vascular resistance approximate
weeks. Pulmonary vascular resistance is st
the first month of life, and cardiac defects
septal defect may not be detected.

The heart is large in relation to body siz
somewhat horizontally and occupies a larg
racic cavity. Growth of the lungs causes t
lower position, and by 7 years of age the
more adult position that is more oblique an
creases in adolescence in conjunction with

At birth ventricular walls are similar i
circulatory demands the left ventricle incre
thinness of the ventricle produces a low s
newborn. The systolic pressure rises after
mates adult levels by puberty. Blood
thicken in response to increased pressures.

Equipment for Assessment of C System

Stethoscope (preferably with a small diap

Preparation

The child may sit or lie. Allow the chi
scope. Listening to the parent's or nurse
hearts is often effective in dispelling anx
Ask the parent or child about heart dis
Inquire whether the child has had diffi

undue fatigue, poor weight gain, weakness, cyanosis, edema, dizziness, squatting, frequent respiratory tract infections, or delayed development. Ask the parent whether the mother had any infection or took medications during pregnancy. Inquire whether the child had problems at birth, such as low birth weight, prematurity, congenital infection, or respiratory difficulty. Inquire about temperament of child and family responses to illness.

Assessment of Heart

Assessment	Findings
Inspection	
Observe the child's body posture.	**Clinical Alert** Squatting is seen in tetralogy of Fallot. Persistent slight hyperextension of the neck in infants may indicate hypoxia.
Observe the child for cyanosis, mottling, and edema.	**Clinical Alert** Cyanosis, pallor, and mottling may indicate heart disease. Edema may be indicative of congestive heart failure. Edema of sacral and periorbital areas is more common in younger children. Edema of the extremities is more common in older children, but in the younger child may be indicative of renal failure.
Observe the child for signs of respiratory difficulty (grunting, costal retractions, flaring of the nares, adventitious chest sounds) and hacking cough.	**Clinical Alert** Respiratory difficulties and congested cough may indicate congestive failure or respiratory infection.
Inspect the child's nailbeds for clubbing, lengthening, or widening.	**Clinical Alert** Clubbing indicates hypoxia.

Assessment	Findings
Examine the anterior chest from an angle. Observe for the symmetry of chest movement, visible pulsations, and diffuse lifts or heaves.	Symmetric chest expansion is normal. In thin children the apical pulse, or point of maximal impulse (PMI), may be seen as a pulsation. **Clinical Alert** Asymmetric chest expansion may signal congestive failure. A systolic heave may indicate right ventricular enlargement.
Palpation	
Using the fingerpads, palpate the anterior chest for the apical pulse or point of maximal impulse (PMI). The location of the PMI is usually felt at the apex of the heart and is found in the fourth intercostal space in children 7 years of age or younger and in the fifth intercostal space in children older than 7 years. The PMI becomes more lateral as the child grows.	The apical pulse normally is palpable in infants and young children. **Clinical Alert** A lower, more lateral PMI may indicate cardiac enlargement. An amplified PMI may indicate anemia, fever, or anxiety.
Fingertips are more useful for detecting pulsations, and the ball of the hand (palmar surface at the base of the fingers) for detecting vibratory thrills or precordial friction rubs. Thrills feel much like the belly of a purring cat.	**Clinical Alert** Rubs are abnormal and should be reported.
Percussion	
Percussion is used to estimate heart size by outlining cardiac borders. It is a difficult technique and has limited usefulness in assessing the	

Assessment	Findings
heart in infants and young children. The location of PMI is a more useful indicator of heart size.	

Auscultation

Assessment	Findings
Using both the bell (for low frequency) and the diaphragm (for high frequency), auscultate for heart sounds. Beginning in the second right intercostal space (aortic area), systematically move the stethoscope from the aortic to the pulmonic area (Figure 15-1). S_2 is best heard at the base of the heart (aortic and pulmonic areas). Move down to Erb's point, and then to the tricuspid and mitral areas. S_1 is heard at the beginning of the apical pulse, which facilitates differentiation of S_1 and S_2. Evaluate the sounds for: Quality (normally S_1 and S_2 are clear and distinct) Rate (synchronous with radial pulse) Intensity (consistent with what would normally be found at each auscultatory point) Rhythm (normally regular)	S_2 is normally loudest in the aortic and pulmonic areas. S_1 and S_2 are equal in intensity at Erb's point. S_1 is loudest in the mitral and tricuspid areas. Sinus arrhythmia is a normal variant in which the rate increases with inspiration and decreases with expiration. **Clinical Alert** S_1 is intensified during fever, exercise, and anemia. Accentuation of S_1 may also indicate mitral stenosis. S_1 that varies in intensity may be indicative of serious arrhythmia and must be reported.
The child should be helped to assume at least two different positions during auscultation.	

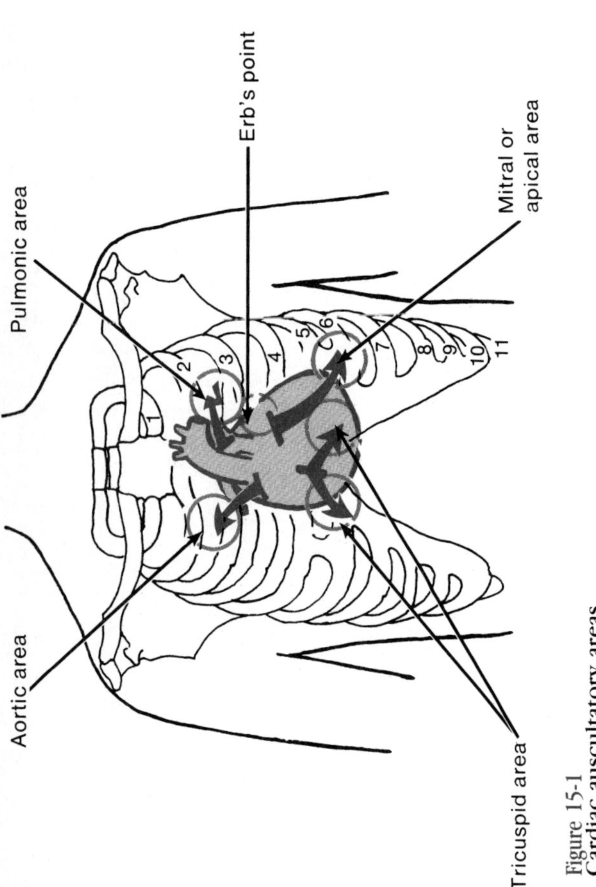

Figure 15-1
Cardiac auscultatory areas.
(From Whaley LF, Wong DL: Nursing care of infants and children, ed 4, St Louis, 1991, Mosby–Year Book.)

Assessment	Findings
Auscultate for additional sounds, such as S_3 and S_4, which are best assessed with the infant or child lying on the left side. Assess for abnormal sounds such as clicks, murmurs, and precordial friction rubs. Murmurs should be evaluated and documented as to:	S_3 is a normal finding.
Location, or auscultatory area in which found	**Clinical Alert** Innocent or nonpathologic murmurs do not increase over time and do not affect the growth of the child. Innocent murmurs are usually systolic (Figure 15-2), low-pitched, musical, and heard at the second and third left interspaces. Innocent murmurs may disappear with change in position.

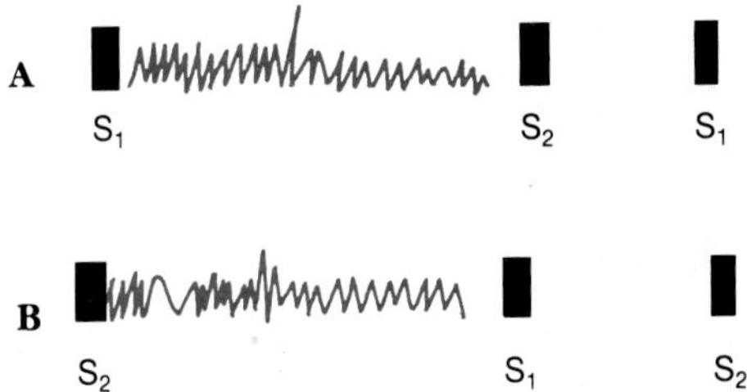

Figure 15-2
Timing of murmurs in S_1-S_2 cycle. A, Systolic murmur. B, Diastolic murmur.

Assessment	Findings
Timing in the S_1-S_2 cycle	Organic murmurs are caused by congenital or acquired heart disease. Murmurs occurring before 3 years of age are usually related to congenital defects, and after 3 years to rheumatic heart disease (see Table 15-2 for a description of murmurs associated with cardiac defects).
Intensity and whether intensity varies with the child's position	
Pitch	
Quality (whether murmur is musical, blowing, or swishing)	
Precordial friction rubs are high-pitched grating sounds that are unaffected by breath-	

Table 15-2 Murmur associated with childhood cardiac defects

Defect	Location	Timing	Intensity	Pitch	Quality
Aortic stenosis	Aortic area	Crescendo effect, occurring between S_1 and S_2	Variable	Medium	Harsh
Pulmonic stenosis	Pulmonic area, third left interspace	Crescendo effect occurring between S_1 and S_2	Variable	Medium	Harsh
Mitral stenosis	Mitral area	Occurs between S_2 and S_1	Variable; may be accentuated by exercise	Low	Rumbling
Aortic regurgitation	Aortic area	Heard between S_2 and S_1; usually a short period follows S_2 before sound begins	Variable; most audible when child leans forward and exhales	High; best heard with diaphragm of stethoscope	Blowing

Mitral regurgitation	Mitral area	Occurs between S_1 and S_2	Variable; unaffected by respiratory cycle	High	Blowing
Ventricular septal defect	Left sternal border, third and fourth interspaces	Heard between S_1 and S_2	Very loud	High	Blowing
Patent ductus arteriosus	Second left interspace	Continuous; louder in late systole (just before S_2); obscures S_2; softer in diastole	Loud	Medium	Harsh
Tetralogy of Fallot	Second and third left interspaces	Heard between S_1 and S_2	Not well transmitted	—	No distinct characteristics

Assessment	Findings
ing patterns. Pleural friction rubs stop when children hold their breath.	Murmurs associated with rheumatic heart disease include those of aortic and mitral stenosis and of aortic and mitral regurgitation. Additional sounds and murmurs must always be described and reported for further evaluation.

Assessment of Vascular System

Assessment of vascular integrity is necessitated by cast application and by other conditions that may impair blood flow. Femoral and dorsal pedal areas should be palpated if cardiac defects are suspected.

Assessment	Findings
Palpate the peripheral arteries for equality, rhythm, and pulse rate.	Normally pulses are palpable, equal in intensity, and even in rhythm.
Palpate the radial pulse. The radial pulse is best felt in children older than 2 years of age.	
Palpate the femoral pulse by applying deep palpation midway between the iliac crest and the symphysis pubis. The child must be in the supine position (Figure 15-3).	**Clinical Alert** Diminution or absence of the femoral pulse may indicate coarctation of the aorta.
Palpate the popliteal pulse by having the child flex the knee (Figure 15-4).	
Palpate the dorsalis pedis pulse along the upper medial aspect of the foot (Figure 15-5).	

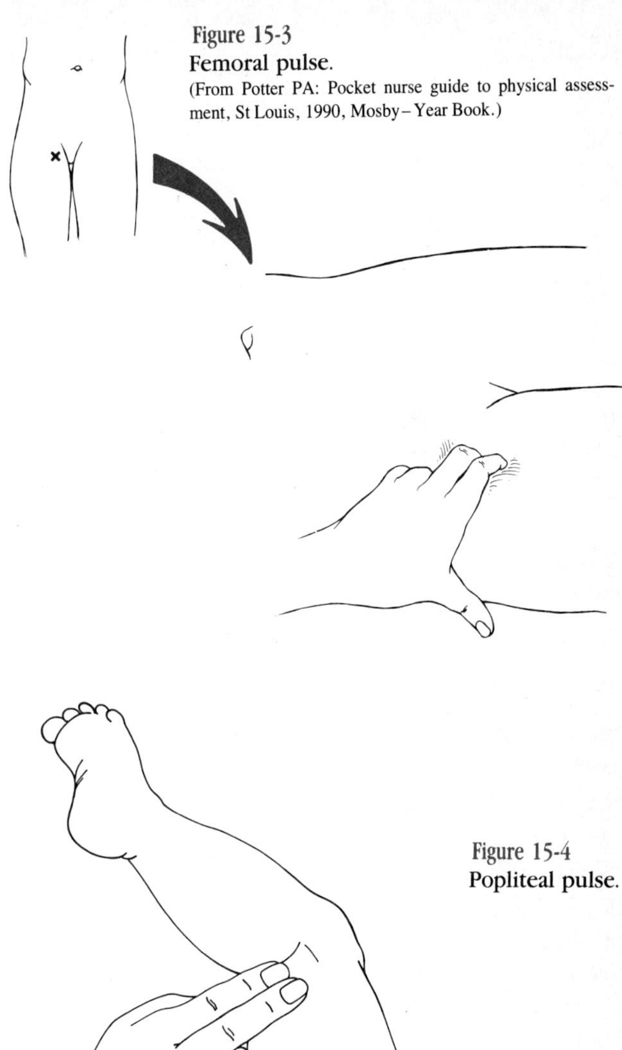

Figure 15-3
Femoral pulse.
(From Potter PA: Pocket nurse guide to physical assessment, St Louis, 1990, Mosby–Year Book.)

Figure 15-4
Popliteal pulse.

Figure 15-5
Dorsalis pedis pulse.

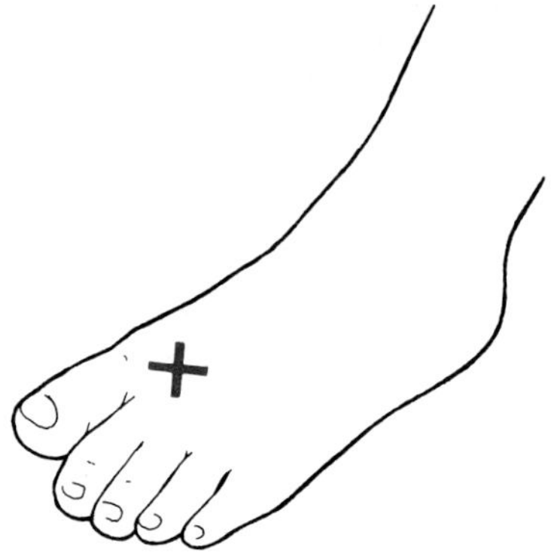

Related Nursing Diagnoses

Activity intolerance: Related to dyspnea and fatigue secondary to decreased cardiac output.

Alteration in nutrition, less than body requirements: Related to nausea; fatigue.

Alteration in tissue perfusion: Peripheral secondary to venous congestion; decreased cardiac output.

Anxiety: Related to difficult breathing; situational crisis.

Family process, alterations in: Related to situational crisis; adjustment to chronic disease.

Fear: Related to progressiveness of condition.

Fluid volume excess: Secondary to decreased cardiac output.

Growth and development, alterations in: Related to activity intolerance; fatigue; social isolation.

Home maintenance, impaired: Related to inability to engage in age-appropriate self-care.

Knowledge deficit: Related to diet; drug therapy; signs and symptoms of complications.

Self-care deficit: Related to activity intolerance; fatigue; breathlessness.

Skin integrity, impairment of: Related to fluid retention.

Sleep pattern, disturbance in: Related to dyspnea secondary to congestive heart failure.

Social interaction, impaired: Related to fatigue; limited mobility.

Abdomen 16

Encased within the abdominal cavity are the organs and structures of the genitourinary, gastrointestinal, and hemopoietic systems. Assessment of the abdomen is really a multiple system assessment and commonly follows assessment of the thorax and lungs.

Lower bowel sounds can be affected by manual manipulation; thus the order of assessment is inspection, auscultation, percussion, and palpation. Because it is sometimes performed as part of the abdominal assessment, assessment of the anus is included in this chapter.

Rationale

The upper gastrointestinal tract is largely inaccessible to the nurse; thus examination of the abdomen primarily involves assessment of lower gastrointestinal and genitourinary structures. Many common childhood disorders involve the gastrointestinal and genitourinary systems, and the function of these systems can also be altered by factors such as surgery, stress, medications, or the hygienic care that the child receives.

Anatomy and Physiology

Gastrointestinal System

The primary functions of the gastrointestinal tract are the digestion and absorption of nutrients and water, elimination of waste products, and secretion of various substances required for digestion.

The liver, located in the right upper quadrant of the abdomen, has several important functions, including biosynthesis of protein; production of blood clotting factors; metabolism of fat, protein, and carbohydrates; production of bile; metabolism of bilirubin; and detoxification.

A primitive gut develops from the endoderm by the third week of gestation. This developing midgut grows so rapidly that by the fourth week of gestation it is too large for the abdominal cavity. Failure of the midgut to rotate and reenter the abdominal cavity at 10 weeks of gestation can produce a variety of disorders, such as omphalocele, and susceptibility to intussusception and bowel obstruction.

The anus arises from a pit invagination of the skin during embryonic development and is the terminal segment of the anal canal. Normally the anal canal is closed by action of the voluntary external sphincter and involuntary internal sphincter muscles. The canal is well supplied by somatic sensory nerves and is sensitive to touch. Externally it is moist and hairless.

Despite the development of the digestive tract in utero, the exchange of nutrients and waste is the function of the placenta. At birth the gastrointestinal tract is still immature and does not fully mature for the first 2 years. Because of this immaturity, many differences exist between the digestive tract of the infant or child and that of the adult. For example, the muscle tone of the lower esophageal sphincter does not assume adult levels until 1 month of age. This lax sphincter muscle tone explains why young infants frequently regurgitate after feedings. Intestinal peristalsis in children is rapid, with emptying time being 2½ to 3 hours in the newborn infant and 3 to 6 hours in older infants and children. Stomach capacity is 10 to 20 ml (0.3 to 0.6 oz) in the neonate, compared with 10 to 200 ml (0.3 to 7.0 oz) in the 2-month-old infant, 1500 ml (50 oz) in the 16-year-old adolescent, and 2000 to 3000 ml (89 to 100 oz) in the adult. The stomach is round and lies somewhat horizontally until 2 years of age. The parietal cells of the stomach do not produce adult levels of hydrochloric acid until 6 months. The gastrocolic reflex, or movement of the contents toward the colon, is rapid in young infants, as evidenced by the frequency of stools. The intestine, which underwent rapid growth in utero, undergoes further growth spurts when the child is 1 to 3 years of age and again at 15 to 16 years. After birth the musculature of the anus develops as the infant becomes more upright. The child then becomes able to voluntarily control defecation.

Genitourinary System

The kidneys lie posteriorly within the upper quadrants of the abdomen. The kidneys regulate fluid and electrolyte levels in the body through filtration, reabsorption, and secretion of water and electrolytes. Water is excreted in the form of urine. The bladder, located below the symphysis pubis, collects the urine for elimination.

The development of the kidneys begins early in gestation but is not complete until near the end of the first year of life. Until the epithelial cells of the nephrons assume a mature flat shape, filtration and absorption are poor. The loop of Henle gradually elongates, which increases the infant's ability to concentrate urine, as seen by fewer wet diapers near the first year of life. Increasing bladder capacity contributes also to decreased frequency of voiding. The infant's bladder capacity is 15 to 20 ml (0.5 to 0.7 oz), compared with 600 to 800 ml (20 to 26.7 oz) in the adult. The size of the kidneys varies with size and age. The kidneys of infants and children are relatively large in comparison with those of adults and are more susceptible to trauma because of their size.

Equipment for Assessment of Abdomen

Warm stethoscope
Warm hands
Short fingernails

Preparation

Ask the parent or child about a family history of gastrointestinal or genitourinary tract disorders and about the child's prenatal history (maternal hydramnios is associated with intestinal atresia). Inquire as to whether the child had imperforate anus, failure to pass meconium, cleft palate or lip, difficulty in feeding, prolonged jaundice, or abdominal wall disorders (for example, omphalocele or hernia), as a neonate. Ask if the child has or has had problems with feeding such as anorexia, vomiting, or regurgitation. If the child has had emesis or regurgitation, determine the time of occurrence, frequency, type (Table 16-1), amount, and force (nonprojectile or projectile). Inquire as to whether the child has or has had pain (frequency, intensity, type, location),

Table 16-1 Types of emesis and related findings

Type of Emesis	Related Findings
Undigested formula or food	Rapid expulsion of stomach contents before digestion has occurred.
Yellow; may smell acidic	Contents originated in stomach.
Dark green (bile stained)	Contents originated below the ampulla of Vater.
Dark brown, foul odor	Emesis produced by intestinal obstruction.
Bright red. Dark red	Bright red signifies fresh bleeding. Dark red signifies old blood or blood altered by gastric secretions.

Table 16-2 Types of stools and related findings

Type of Stool	Related Findings
Soft or liquid	Indicative of breast-feeding.
Light yellow, pasty. Soft or pasty green	Common in formula-fed babies. Stool has been exposed to air for some time, and oxidation has occurred.
Liquid or watery green	Diarrhea.
Black	May indicate that the child is receiving iron or bismuth preparations or has gastric or duodenal bleeding.
Gray or clay colored	Intestinal atresia may be present.
Undigested food in stool	Common in infants who are unable to completely digest foods, such as corn and carrots.
Currant jelly stool (blood and mucus)	Indicative of intussusception.
Ribbon-like	Indicative of Hirschsprung's disease.
Frothy, foul smelling	Indicative of cystic fibrosis.

itching (location), swelling, tendency to bruise, thirst, dry mouth, unexplained fever, food allergies, sensitivity to diapers, or alterations in bowel movements or in urinary elimination patterns. If there is a problem with bowel movements, inquire as to the frequency, amount, consistency, quality, and color of stool (Table 16-2). If there are alterations in the pattern of urinary elimination, determine what they are and when they began. If problems with urination or bowel movements occur in toddlers, explore what these problems mean to parents. In the school-aged child who experiences recurrent abdominal pain, explore possible stressors and responses to stressors.

It is important that the child be relaxed during abdominal examination, particularly during palpation. Flexing the child's head or hips helps to relax abdominal muscles. Flexing the child's knees permits greater visibility of the anal area. Talking and playing with the child also assists in examination. Most children are ticklish, so briefly place a hand flat on the abdomen before beginning the examination. A very ticklish child can be assisted by placing the child's hand over the nurse's during palpation.

Assessment of Abdomen

Assessment	Findings
Inspection	
Inspect the contour of the abdomen while the infant or child is standing and while lying supine.	A pot-bellied or prominent abdomen is normal until puberty, related to lordosis of the spine. The abdomen appears flat when the child is supine. **Clinical Alert** An especially protuberant abdomen may suggest fluid retention, tumor, organomegaly (enlarged organ), or ascites.

Assessment	Findings
	A large abdomen, with thin limbs and wasted buttocks, suggests severe malnutrition and may be seen in children with celiac disease or cystic fibrosis. A depressed abdomen is indicative of dehydration or high abdominal obstruction. A midline protrusion from the xiphoid process to the umbilicus or the symphysis pubis is indicative of diastasis recti abdominis.
Inspect the color and condition of the skin of the abdomen. Note the presence of scars and ecchymoses.	**Clinical Alert** Yellowish coloration may suggest jaundice. Silver lines (striae) are indicative of obesity or of fluid retention. Scars may indicate previous surgery. Ecchymoses of soft tissue areas can indicate abuse.
Inspect the abdomen for movement by standing at eye level to the abdomen.	**Clinical Alert** Visible peristaltic waves nearly always indicate intestinal obstruction, and in the infant younger than 2 months indicate pyloric stenosis. Failure of the abdomen and thorax to move synchronously may indicate peritonitis (if the abdomen does not move) or pulmonary disease (if the thorax does not move).

Assessment	Findings
Inspect the umbilicus for color, discharge, odor, inflammation, and herniation.	**Clinical Alert** A bluish umbilicus is indicative of intraabdominal hemorrhage. A nodular umbilicus is indicative of tumor. Protrusion of the umbilicus is indicative of herniation. Umbilical hernias protrude more noticeably with crying and coughing. Palpate the umbilicus to estimate the size of the opening. Drainage from the umbilicus may indicate infection or a patent urachus.
Auscultation	
Auscultate for bowel sounds by pressing both the bell and the diaphragm of the stethoscope *firmly* against the abdomen. Listen in all four quadrants (Figure 16-1) and count the bowel sounds in each quadrant for 1 full minute. Before deciding that bowel sounds are absent, the nurse must listen for a minimum of 5 minutes. Bowel sounds can be stimulated, if present, by stroking the abdomen with a fingernail.	Normal bowel sounds occur every 10 to 30 seconds and are heard as gurgles, clicks, and growls. **Clinical Alert** High-pitched tinkling sounds are indicative of diarrhea, gastroenteritis, or obstruction. Absence of bowel sounds may indicate peritonitis or paralytic ileus.
Percussion	
Using indirect percussion, systematically percuss all areas of the abdomen.	Dullness or flatness is normally found along the right costal margin (Figure 16-1) and 1 to 3 cm (0.4 to 1.4 in) below the costal margin of the liver.

Assessment	Findings
	Dullness above the symphysis pubis may be indicative of a full bladder in a young child and is normal.
	Tympany is normally heard throughout the rest of the abdomen.
	Clinical Alert
	Areas of unexpected dullness or flatness may be indicative of large masses of feces.
	If liver dullness extends lower than expected, an enlarged liver may be suspected.

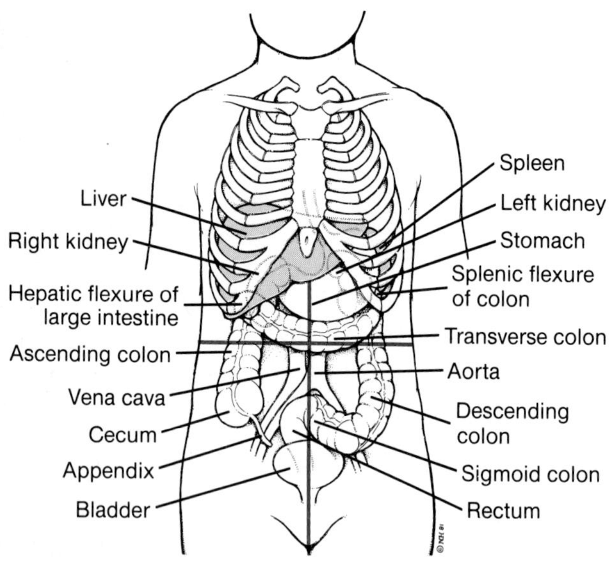

Figure 16-1

Anatomic landmarks of abdomen.

(From Whaley LF, Wong DL: Nursing care of infants and children, ed 4, St Louis, 1991, Mosby–Year Book.)

Assessment	Findings

Palpation

If the child complains of pain in an abdominal area, palpate that area last.

Using superficial palpation, assess the abdomen for tenderness, superficial lesions, muscle tone, turgor (pinch the skin into a fold), and cutaneous hyperesthesia (pick up a fold of skin but do not pinch). Superficial palpation is performed by placing the hand on the abdomen and applying light pressure with the fingertips. Note areas of tenderness. *Visceral* pain, arising from organs, is dull and poorly localized. *Somatic* pain, arising from the walls and the linings of the abdominal cavity, is sharp and well defined. Do not ask, "Does this hurt?" The child, eager to please, may say yes.

Clinical Alert

A child's withdrawal or tense facial expression may be indicative of apprehension or pain.

Pain on picking up a fold of abdominal skin is indicative of cutaneous hyperesthesia, which may be found with peritonitis.

Perform deep palpation, either by placing one hand on top of the other or by supporting posterior structures with one hand while palpating anterior structures with the other. Palpate from the lower quadrants upward so that an enlarged liver can be detected.

Discomfort in the epigastrium on deep palpation is related to pressure over the aorta.

The spleen tip may be palpated 1 to 2 cm (0.4 to 0.8 in) below the left costal margin during inspiration in infants and young children and is felt as a soft, thumb-shaped object.

Assessment	Findings
	The liver may be palpated below the right costal margin during inspiration in infants and young children. The liver edge is firm and smooth.
	Kidneys are rarely palpable except in neonates.
	The sigmoid colon may be palpable as a tender sausage-shaped mass in the left lower quadrant. The cecum may be palpated as a soft mass in the right lower quadrant.

Clinical Alert

Tenderness in the lower quadrants may indicate feces, gastroenteritis, pelvic infection, or tumor.

Tenderness in the left upper quadrant may indicate splenic enlargement or intussusception.

Tenderness in the right upper quadrant may be related to hepatitis or an enlarged liver.

Tenderness in the right lower quadrant or around the umbilicus may indicate appendicitis. *Rebound tenderness* indicates appendicitis and may be elicited by applying pressure distal to where the child states there is pain. Pain is experienced in the original area of tenderness when pressure is *released*. An enlarged spleen is indicative of infection or blood disease.

Assessment	Findings
	An enlarged liver is found with infection and blood dycrasias. Enlarged kidneys may indicate tumor or hydronephrosis. Intestinal masses may be indicative of tumors or stool. A distended bladder may be palpable above the symphysis pubis.
Further assess for peritoneal irritation by performing the psoas muscle test. This test can be performed in a cooperative older child if the nurse is assessing for appendicitis. Have the child flex the right leg at the hip and knee while you apply downward pressure. Normally, no pain is felt.	**Clinical Alert** Pain suggests appendicitis.
Palpate for an inguinal hernia by sliding the little finger into the external inguinal canal at the base of the scrotum.	**Clinical Alert** Report the presence of inguinal hernia. An inguinal hernia is felt as a bulge when the child laughs or cries. Inguinal hernia is more common in boys.
Palpate for a femoral hernia by locating the femoral pulse. Place the index finger on the pulse and the middle ring finger medially against the skin. The ring finger is over the area where the herniation occurs.	**Clinical Alert** Report the presence of femoral hernia. A femoral hernia is felt or seen as a small anterior mass. Femoral hernia is more commonly found in girls.

Assessment of Anal Area

Assessment	Findings
With the child prone, inspect the buttocks and thighs. Examine the skin around the anal area for redness and rash.	**Clinical Alert** Asymmetry of the buttocks and thigh folds is indicative of congenital hip dysplasia. Redness and rash may indicate inadequate cleaning after bowel movements, infrequent changing of diapers, or irritation from diarrhea.
Examine the anus for marks, fissures (tears in the mucosa), hemorrhoids (dark protrusions), prolapse (moist tube-like protrusion), polyps (bright red protrusions), and skin tags.	The anus usually appears moist and hairless. **Clinical Alert** Scratch marks may indicate itching, which can be indicative of pinworm infestation. Fissures may be indicative of passage of hard stools. Defecation may be accompanied by bleeding if fissures are present. Bleeding can also accompany polyps, intussusception, gastric and peptic ulcers, esophageal varices, ulcerative colitis, infectious diseases, and Meckel's diverticulum. Rectal prolapse is indicative of difficult defecation and frequently accompanies untreated cystic fibrosis. Skin tags can be indicative of polyps and are usually benign.

Assessment	Findings
Stroke the anal area to elicit the anal reflex.	The anus should contract quickly. **Clinical Alert** A slow reflex may indicate a disorder of the pyramidal tract.

Related Nursing Diagnoses

Anxiety: Related to knowledge deficit; discomfort.

Bowel elimination, alteration in: Constipation related to altered bowel motility; diet.

Bowel elimination, alteration in: Diarrhea related to altered bowel motility; diet.

Comfort, alterations in: Pain related to altered bowel motility; bowel distention; bladder distention; loss of skin integrity; pruritus.

Family processes, alterations in: Related to skill or knowledge deficit; stress.

Fluid volume deficit: Related to excess fluid loss; limited intake; increased metabolic rate.

Fluid volume excess: Secondary to liver disorders; renal disorders.

Health maintenance, alterations in: Related to knowledge deficit.

Knowledge deficit: Related to disease process; dietary alterations; hygienic needs.

Parenting, alterations in: Related to skill deficit.

Skin integrity, impairment of: Related to pruritus; knowledge deficit; incontinence (urine or feces).

Urinary elimination, alterations in patterns of: Related to inflammation; infection; retention; artificial drainage system.

Lymphatic System 17

The lymphatic system includes the lymph nodes, spleen, thymus, and bone marrow. The superficial lymph nodes and the spleen are accessible for assessment and are discussed in this chapter. Assessment of the lymphatic system is often integrated with assessment of the neck, breast, and abdomen.

Rationale

The most common causes of visible lymphoid activity are infection and neoplasms. Infection is the most common cause of lumps in children's necks. An understanding of which areas are drained by the nodes is useful in further assessment of present or past infections. Detection of enlarged nodes and an enlarged spleen can be critical to the early diagnosis and treatment of serious disorders.

Anatomy and Physiology

The lymphoid system is a system of lymph fluid, collecting ducts, and tissues. Although the specific functions of lymphoid tissue are still not fully understood, the system is thought to play an important role in the production of lymphocytes and antibodies and in phagocytosis. The system also transports lymph fluids, microorganisms, and protein back to the cardiovascular system and absorbs fat and fat-soluble substances from the intestine.

Lymph enters open-ended ducts called capillaries. The capillaries form larger collecting ducts, which drain into tissue centers or nodes. Lymph from the nodes eventually drains into the venous system by way of even larger ducts.

Lymph nodes, the most numerous element in the lymphatic system, rarely occur singly, but usually in chains or clusters. The lymph nodes that are closer to the center of the body are usually smaller; thus cervical nodes are larger than axillary nodes. The spleen is composed of lymphoid and reticuloendothelial cells. It is found under the ribs in the upper left quadrant of the abdomen. The amount of lymphoid tissue and the size of the lymph nodes vary with age. Infants have a small amount of palpable lymphatic tissue, which gradually increases until middle childhood, when the volume of lymphatic tissue reaches its peak. By mid-adolescence the volume of lymphatic tissue begins to diminish, until it reaches the adult level of 2% to 3% of total body weight. Children are more likely to develop generalized adenopathy in response to disease, and even mild infections result in swollen nodes or "swollen glands."

Equipment for Assessment of Lymphatic System

Ruler

Preparation

Inquire about recent contacts with persons with infectious diseases. Ask if the child has been experiencing weakness, easy fatigability, fever, bruising, or chronic or recurrent infection. Ask if there is a family history of blood disorders or cancer.

Assessment of Lymph Nodes

Assessment	Findings
Using the distal portion of the fingers and gentle but firm circular motions, palpate the head, neck, axillae, and groin to detect enlarged lymph nodes (Figure 17-1). Note the color, size, location, temperature, consistency, and tenderness of enlarged nodes. Tender nodes should be assessed last. Measure enlarged nodes.	Small (less than 1 cm, or ½ in), movable, nontender nodes are normal in young children. **Clinical Alert** Nodes that are enlarged because of infection are firm, warm, fluctuant, and movable and their borders are diffuse. Redness may overlie nodes that are enlarged because of infection.

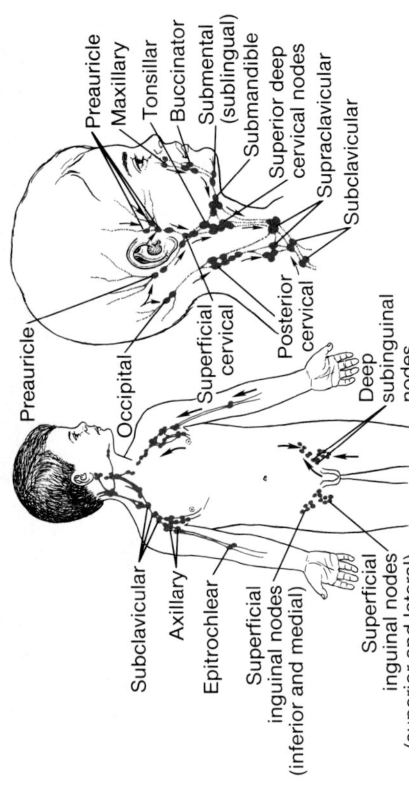

Figure 17-1
Location of lymph nodes and direction of lymph flow.
(From Whaley LF, Wong DL: Nursing care of infants and children, ed 4, St Louis, 1991, Mosby–Year Book.)

Assessment	Findings
To palpate nodes in the areas anterior and posterior to the sternocleidomastoid muscle, move the fingertips against the muscle.	Enlargement of the preauricular, mastoid, and deep cervical nodes may indicate infection of the ear.
To palpate nodes in the head and neck, have the child flex the head forward or bend toward side being examined.	Enlargement of nodes in the jaw may signify infections of the tongue or mouth.
To palpate nodes in the axillae, roll the tissues against the chest wall and muscles of the axillae. Have the child hold the arms in a relaxed, slightly abducted position at the sides.	Enlargement of nodes in the supraclavicular region is often indicative of metastases from the lungs or abdominal structures.
To palpate nodes in the inguinal area, place the child supine.	Nodes enlarged as a result of cancer are usually nontender, fixed, hard, of variable size, and matted. No discoloration is present.
	Enlarged nodes may also be indicative of metabolic disorders, hypersensitivity reactions, and primary hematopoietic disorders.

Assessment of Spleen

Assessment	Findings
With the child supine, place one hand under the child's back and the other hand on the left upper quadrant of the child's abdomen. Ask the child to "Suck in your breath." The spleen tip can be felt during inspiration on deep palpation.	The spleen can be palpated 1 to 2 cm (0.4 to 0.8 in) below the left costal margin in infants and children. **Clinical Alert** A spleen that extends more than 2 cm (0.8 in) below the costal margin may be indicative of leukemia or thalassemia major.

Related Nursing Diagnoses

Activity intolerance: Related to weakness; fatigue.

Coping, ineffective family: Compromised related to situational-crisis; knowledge deficit.

Hyperthermia: Related to infection.

Injury, potential for: Related to presence of infective organisms.

Nutrition, alterations in: Less than body requirements related to increased metabolism.

Reproductive System 18

Assessment of the reproductive system in infants and children includes inspection of the external genitalia. Examination of internal genitalia is performed by nurses specially prepared in this skill.

Rationale

Examination of the external genitalia enables screening for common disorders that arise from prenatal development and influences. Examination enables the nurse to detect infections that require further evaluation. Assessment of the reproductive system frequently provides a beginning point for teaching and discussion related to sexuality and hygiene.

Anatomy and Physiology

Female Genitalia

The female genitalia includes the external and internal sex organs. The external sex organs, or vulva, include the mons pubis, a fatty pad overlying the symphysis pubis (Figure 18-1); the labia majora, rounded folds of adipose tissue extending down and back from the mons pubis; the labia minora, two thinner folds of skin medial to the labia majora; and the clitoris, an erectile body situated at the anterior end of the labia minora. The labia minora are homologous to the male scrotum, and the clitoris to the male penis. Underlying the labia minora is a boat-shaped area termed the vestibule. At the posterior end of the vestibule is the vaginal opening, or introitus, which may be partially obscured by the hymen, a vascular mucous membrane. The perineum is the area between the vaginal opening and the anus. The urethral opening, or urinary meatus, lies between the vaginal opening and the clitoris. On either side of the urethral opening can be seen Skene's glands, or the paraurethral ducts. Bartholin's glands, which secrete lubricating fluid during intercourse, are situated on either side of the vaginal opening, but the openings to the glands usually cannot be seen.

The vagina is a hollow tube extending upward and backward between the urethra and the rectum. The cervix joins the vagina, which has a slitlike opening, termed the external os, that provides an opening between the uterus and the endocervical canal. The uterus is a muscular pear-shaped organ suspended above the bladder. In the prepubescent girl the uterus is 2.5 to 3.5 cm (1 to 1.5 in) long, compared with 6 to 8 cm (2.4 to 3.2 in) in the mature woman. The uterine, or fallopian, tubes extend from the

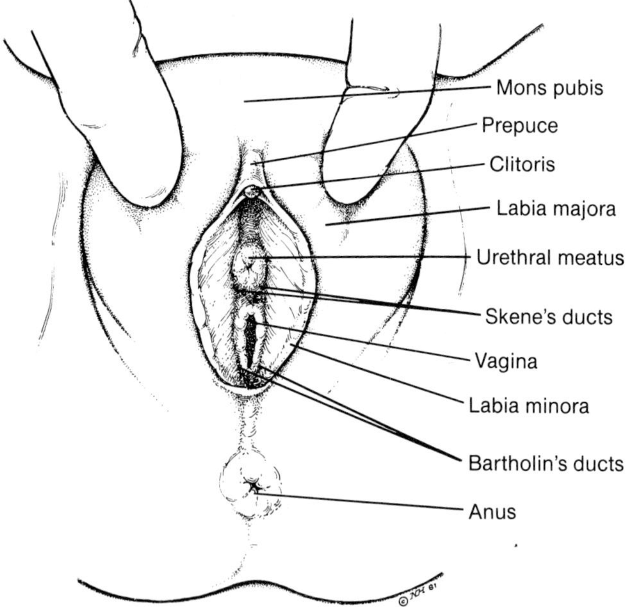

Figure 18-1
External female genitalia.
(From Whaley LF, Wong DL: Nursing care of infants and children, ed 4, St Louis, 1991, Mosby–Year Book.)

uterus to the ovaries and produce a passageway in which ova and sperm meet.

Male Genitalia

The external male genitalia includes the penis and scrotum. The penis consists of a shaft and a glans (Figure 18-2). The shaft is formed primarily of erectile tissue. The glans is a cone-shaped structure at the end of the penis and contains both erectile and sensory tissue. The corona is the crownlike area where the glans arises from the shaft. A loose fold of skin, termed the prepuce or foreskin, overlies the glans. This skin is removed during circumcision. The urethra is within the penile shaft, with the slitlike urethral meatus located slightly centrally at the tip of the glans.

The scrotum is a loose, wrinkled sac located at the base of the penis. The scrotum has two compartments, each of which contains a testis, epididymis, and parts of the vas deferens. The testes, epididymis, and vas deferens are considered internal male sex organs.

The testes are ovoid and somewhat rubbery. The testes in the infant are 1.5 cm (0.6 in) long. Testicular length remains virtu-

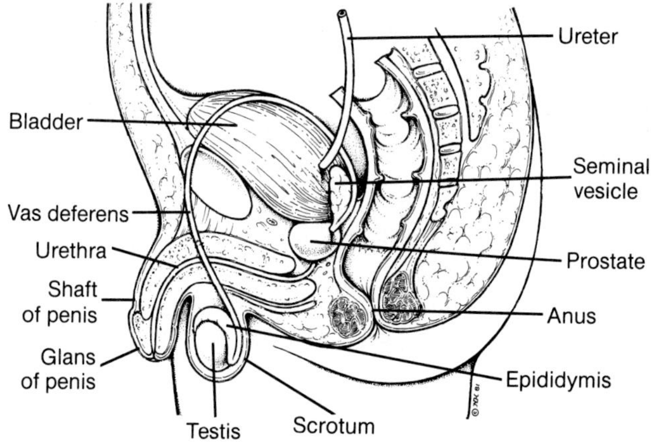

Figure 18-2
Male genitalia.
(From Whaley LF, Wong DL: Nursing care of infants and children, ed 4, St Louis, 1991, Mosby–Year Book.)

ally unchanged until puberty, when the testes gradually enlarge to the adult length of 4 to 5 cm (1.6 to 2 in). The left testis lies slightly lower than the right. Primary functions of the testis are sperm and hormone production. During ejaculation sperm drain into the epididymis, and then into the vas deferens before passing into the urethra.

The genetic sex type of the embryo begins during cell division, when X and Y chromosomes are distributed. Initially, internal and external genitalia are not differentiated (Figure 18-3, *A*). External differentiation begins by about the seventh week of gestation. Under the influence of androgens, enlargement and fusion of primitive urogenital structures occurs and male genitalia are formed (Figure 18-3, *B*). The testes descend from the abdominal cavity at between 7 and 9 months of gestation. If the tube that precedes their descent fails to close, an indirect inguinal hernia is produced.

The male reproductive system remains unchanged until maturity. Testicular enlargement is a visible sign of sexual matura-

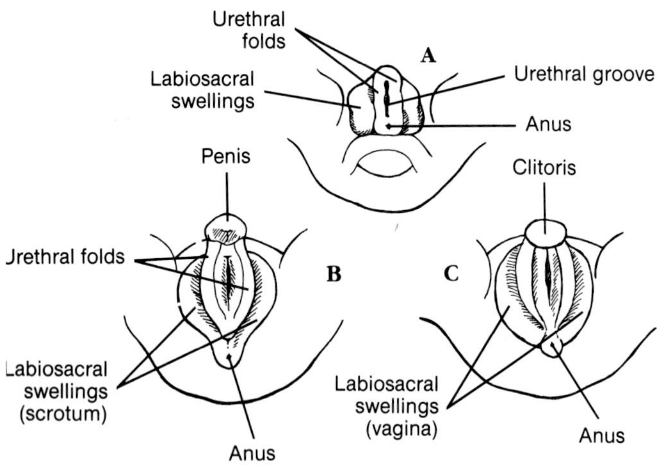

Figure 18-3
Initial stages in embryonic genital development. A, Undifferentiated stage. **B,** Initial differentiation of external genitalia in male embryo. **C,** Initial differentiation of external genitalia in female embryo.

tion, which may begin by 10 years of age. Accompanying the initial increase in testicular size are a coarsening, reddening, and wrinkling of the scrotal sacs and the growth of a few pubic hairs (the child has no pubic hair). Height and weight increase, and hair growth appears on the face about 2 years after the appearance of pubic hair. During further development the penis enlarges, the voice changes, and body odor appears. The genital skin continues to pigment and the external sex organs continue to enlarge until full maturation is reached. At maturity pubic hair covers the symphysis pubis and medial aspects of the thighs. Reproductive capability accompanies sexual maturity, which is accomplished between 14 and 18 years of age.

In the embryo, development of female genitalia involves shrinkage and minimal fusion of primitive urogenital structures (Figure 18-3, *C*). Primordial follicles are formed during the sixth month of gestation, but must wait until puberty for further development. Breast development is usually the first sign of sexual maturation, although growth of pubic hair may precede breast enlargement. The initial pubic hair, located at the sides of the labia, is fine. Gradually the hair coarsens, and covers the sides of the labia and the perianal area at full maturation. Internal and external sex organs enlarge. The onset of menstruation provides observable evidence of reproductive maturation (Figure 18-4).

Equipment for Assessment of Reproductive System

Glove for pelvic examination
Drape
Speculum

Preparation

A casual, matter-of-fact approach facilitates examination of the reproductive system. Much of the examination can be accomplished during assessment of the abdomen and anus in the infant and younger child. Inform parents and child of results of the finding as the assessment progresses, as this helps to relieve anxiety. A child other than an infant should be adequately covered at all times with clothing or a drape. The first pelvic examination is usually performed when the female child is 16 to 18 years old or

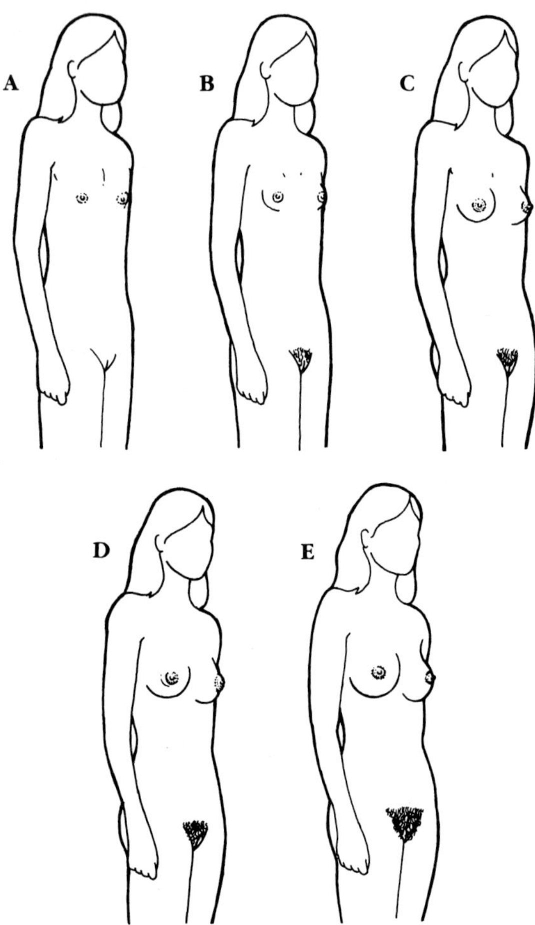

Figure 18-4
Stages in development of female breasts and female pubic hair. **A,** Prepubescent. Papilla elevates. No pubic hair. **B,** Breast bud stage. Breast and papilla elevate as a small mound. Areola enlarges. Sparse long, straight pubic hair. **C,** Breast and areola enlarge further. Heavier, coarser pubic hair. **D,** Areola and papilla project from breast. Pubic hair similar to that in adult but covers smaller area. **E,** Mature form. Papilla elevates but areola recedes into breast. Pubic hair is adult in distribution and quantity.

as soon as she becomes sexually active, when there is a history of trauma or abuse, when there is vaginal discharge or menstrual difficulty, or at the adolescent's request.

Inquire whether the female child has or has had itching, pain on urination, or vaginal discharge. If the girl is older, inquire whether menses have commenced, the date of the last menstrual period, and if the child knows how or is practicing breast self-examination.

Inquire whether the male child has or has had decreased urination, forced urination, a strong urinary stream, or pain on voiding, or any discharge or drip from the penis.

Assessment of Female Breasts

Assessment is accomplished with the adolescent sitting with arms at her sides. Because the adolescent must disrobe to the waist, ensure that the room is warm. Privacy is essential. Tell the adolescent that you are going to examine her breasts. A gentle matter-of-fact approach assists in putting her at ease. If the adolescent is unfamiliar with breast self-examination, this is a good opportunity to explain what is being done and to encourage her to imitate the examination maneuvers. Adolescents may be too embarrassed to touch their breasts, and the nurse's approach should vary with the patient's degree of psychologic comfort.

Assessment	Findings
Inspect the breasts. Note their size, contour, symmetry, and color.	Contour and size of the breasts and changes in the areola indicate sexual maturity. Some difference in size of the breasts is usually normal. One breast may develop before the other, and the adolescent may need reassurance that this is normal. **Clinical Alert** Breast development before 8 years of age may be normal but requires careful assessment.

Assessment	Findings
	Delayed breast development (none by age 13 years) should be evaluated along with the development of secondary sexual characteristics. Dimpling and alterations in the contour of the breast may be indicative of cancer. Redness may signal infection.
Inspect the nipple and areola. Note their color, size, shape, and the presence and color of any discharge.	The color, size, and shape of the nipple and areola provide information about sexual maturity. **Clinical Alert** Flattening of the nipple in a more mature adolescent or edema of the nipple or areola may indicate the presence of cancer. Discharge is an abnormal finding and may be due to a number of causes, most of them nonmalignant. It should be referred to a physician.
Have the adolescent place her arms above her head, and then on her hips. These maneuvers help to accentuate dimpling or retraction that may be missed.	
Palpate the breast tissue with the patient supine and with her hands behind her neck. If breasts are large, place a pillow under the patient's	Normal young breast tissue has firm elasticity. The stimulation of examination may cause erection of the nipple and wrinkling of the areola.

Assessment	Findings
shoulder on the side that is to be examined. This distributes the breast tissue more evenly. Begin palpation on the breast opposite the one with a reported mass so that comparison is more reliable. Use the pads of the first three fingers to gently compress the breast tissue against the chest wall. Using a rotary motion, systematically palpate the entire breast, including the periphery, areola, nipple, and tail. During palpation note consistency of tissues and areas of tenderness.	**Clinical Alert** Fixed hard nodules with unclear borders may indicate cancer.
Palpate abnormal masses and note their location (by quadrant), size (in centimeters or inches), shape (round, discoid, irregular), consistency, tenderness, mobility, discreteness (well-circumscribed or not).	

Assessment of Female Genitalia

Assessment is best accomplished with the child supine. Encouraging the child to keep her heels together provides distraction.

Assessment	Findings
Inspect the mons pubis for hair. Note color, quality, quantity, and distribution of hair, if present.	Soft, downy, hair along the labia majora signals early sexual maturation.
	In the mature woman, pubic hair forms an inverted triangle.

Assessment	Findings
Inspect the labia majora and labia minora for size, color, skin integrity, and masses.	Labia should appear pink and moist. **Clinical Alert** Redness and swelling of labia may indicate infection, masturbation, or sexual abuse. Fusion of labia may be indicative of male scrotum. Labial adhesions may be seen in infants. Blisters and pimples may indicate venereal disease. Venereal disease in the young child is a sign of sexual abuse. Urogenital abnormalities are found in infants born to mothers who used cocaine prenatally.
Note the size of the clitoris.	**Clinical Alert** A clitoris larger than normal may be indicative of labioscrotal fusion.
Inspect urethral and vaginal openings for edema, redness, and discharge. Palpate for Skene's and Bartholin's glands.	Skene's and Bartholin's glands are normally not palpable. **Clinical Alert** Redness of the urethra may indicate urethritis. Redness and foul-smelling discharge from the vagina may indicate a foreign body, infection, sexual abuse, or pinworms. A white, cheesy, discharge from the vagina is indicative of a candidal infection.

Assessment	Findings
	If Bartholin's or Skene's glands are palpable, infection or cysts may be present. Refer the child for further examination if a vaginal opening cannot be seen.

Assessment of Male Genitalia

Assessment	Findings
Inspect the penis for size, color, and skin integrity. Note whether the child is circumcised. If uncircumcised and older than 3 years of age, attempt to retract the foreskin. Do not forcibly attempt to retract the foreskin.	An obese child may appear to have a small penis because of overlying skin folds. The foreskin is normally adherent in children younger than 3 years. **Clinical Alert** A penis that is large in relation to the child's stage of development may suggest precocious puberty or testicular cancer. An abnormally small penis may be indicative of a clitoris. A round, dark red, painless sore is a syphilitic chancre and should be reported. Condyloma acuminatum, or warts, is a venereal disease and may indicate sexual activity in an adolescent or sexual abuse in a young child. A foreskin that cannot be easily retracted in a child older than 3 years may be indicative of phimosis.

Assessment	Findings
Inspect the urinary meatus for shape, placement, discharge, and ulceration. If possible, note the strength and steadiness of the urinary stream.	The urinary meatus is normally *slightly* ventral at the tip of the penis and slitlike. **Clinical Alert** A urinary meatus that is ventral is called hypospadias. A meatus that is dorsal is called epispadias. A round meatus may be indicative of meatal stenosis related to repeated infections.
Inspect the quality, quantity, and distribution of pubic hair. Inspect the scrotum for color, size, symmetry, edema, masses, and lesions. Palpate the testes by holding a finger over the inguinal canal while palpating the scrotal sac. Cold, touch, exercise, and stimulation cause the testes to ascend higher into the pelvic cavity. This can be prevented by palpating the inguinal canal or by having the child sit tailor fashion.	A prepubertal boy normally does not have pubic hair (Figure 18-5). The left testis is lower than the right. A testes should be present in each sac, freely movable, smooth, equal in size and about 1.5 cm (0.8 in) until puberty. **Clinical Alert** The absence of a testis in the scrotal sac may indicate temporary ascent of the testis into the pelvic cavity or an undescended testicle. Reassess. If testes still cannot be felt, refer the child if older than 3 years. Before 3 years the testicle may descend without intervention. If both testes are undescended this may indicate pseudohermaphroditism, especially if hypospadias or a small penis is also present.

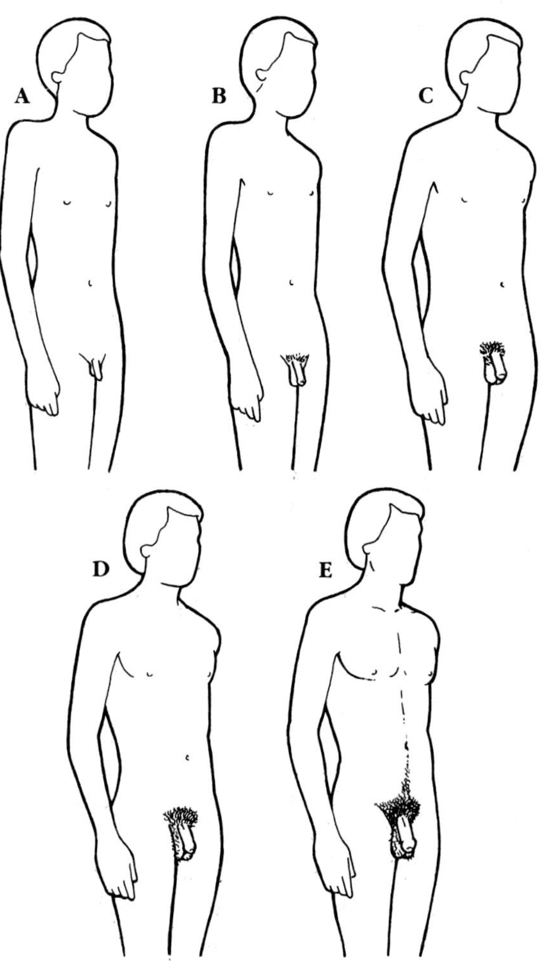

Figure 18-5
Stages in development of male genitalia. **A,** Prepubescent. Genitals are the same as those in childhood. **B,** Scrotum and testes enlarge. Scrotal skin reddens. Downy, straight hair grows at base of penis. **C,** Penis, scrotum, and testes enlarge. Hair becomes curly, coarser. **D,** Penis enlarges further. Scrotum darkens. Hair similar to that of an adult but covers smaller area. **E,** Genitals and hair are adultlike.

Related Nursing Diagnoses

Communication, impaired: Verbal related to fear; body changes; knowledge deficit.

Coping, ineffective family: Related to family history of sexual abuse.

Family process, alteration in: Related to sexual maturation.

Fear: Related to knowledge deficit.

Infection: Related to increased sexual contact.

Knowledge deficit: Related to normal development; safe sexual practices; breast self-examination.

Self-care deficit: Related to hygiene in uncircumcised boys; hygiene during menses.

Self-concept: Disturbances in body image, self-esteem, role performance, personal identity related to sexual changes.

Sexuality patterns, altered: Related to sexual maturation; emerging sexual identity.

Skin integrity, impairment of: Related to infection; discharge.

Musculoskeletal System 19

The nurse can obtain a great deal of data about the musculoskeletal system by watching the child walk, sit, and carry on various activities during other portions of the health assessment. Specific assessments aid in screening for childhood disorders such as clubfoot, congenital hip dislocation, and scoliosis.

Rationale

Movement is so much a part of a child's activities that it is important to screen for disorders that may affect a child's socialization, exercise patterns, and ability to engage in self-care. Early diagnosis and intervention in disorders such as congenital hip dislocation can possibly prevent more exhaustive treatment as the child grows older.

Anatomy and Physiology

The musculoskeletal system provides support for the body and enables movement. The musculoskeletal system is composed of bones, muscles, tendons, ligaments, cartilage, and joints.

The skeleton arises from mesoderm. At birth the epiphyses of most bones are made of hyaline cartilage. Shortly after birth, secondary ossification centers appear in the epiphyses. The epiphyses ossify, except for the epiphyseal plate, which separates the epiphyses and the diaphyses. The epiphyseal plate is replaced by bone until only the epiphyseal line remains. When the epiphyses are completely ossified, no further bone lengthening occurs.

Muscle fibers are developed by the fourth or fifth month of gestation. The number of muscle fibers remains constant throughout life. Muscle growth is accomplished by increase in the size of the fibers. Muscle mass increases from one fourth of total body weight at birth to one sixth of total body weight at adolescence.

Preparation

Inquire whether the infant sustained trauma or injury at birth. Inquire whether there is a family history of bone or joint disorders and whether the child has experienced delays in gross or fine motor development, trauma, joint stiffness and swelling, or pain. If the child has or has had pain, it is important to determine the location, type, intensity, and time of occurrence of the pain. Sharp pain that lessens during rest may indicate injury. Constant dull pain that awakens the child might be indicative of tumor or infection.

Minimal clothing assists with assessment of the spine.

Assessment of Musculoskeletal System

Assessment	Findings
If the child is able to walk, observe the gait. Note the presence of casts and braces.	Infants and toddlers tend to walk bowlegged. A wide-based gait is normal in the infant and toddler. **Clinical Alert** Limping may be indicative of congenital dislocation of one hip. If both hips are involved, the child has a waddling gait. (Table 19-1 lists further indications of congenital hip dislocation.) Limping is also indicative of scoliosis, Legg-Calvé-Perthes disease, infection of the joints of the lower extremities, or a slipped capital femoral epiphyses.

Assessment	Findings
	Weight bearing on the toes (pes equinus) and short heel cords are indicative of muscular disease or cerebral palsy.
Observe the curve of the infant's or child's spine and note the symmetry of the hips and shoulders. Test for scoliosis by having the child bend forward at the waist and observing the child from front, back, and side.	The spine is normally rounded in the infant younger than 3 months. A lumbar curve forms at 12 to 18 months. Lumbar lordosis is normal in young children. **Clinical Alert** Kyphosis (hunchback) indicates wedge-shaped or collapsed vertebrae secondary to myelomeningocele, spinal tumors, Sheuermann's disease, or tuberculosis of the spine. Kyphosis may also be indicative of habitual slouching. The persistence of lateral curvature of the spine is indicative of scoliosis. If the child can voluntarily correct the curve or if it disappears when the child is recumbent, the curve may be functional. A persistent curve, accompanied by unequal height of the shoulders and iliac crests when the child is standing erect and asymmetric elevation of the scapula when the child is leaning forward (Figure 19-1) are indicative of structural scoliosis.
Note the mobility of the spine, especially the cervical spine.	No resistance or pain should be felt when the child bends or when the neck is flexed or moved from side to side.

Assessment	Findings
	Clinical Alert Pain, crying, or resistance when the neck is flexed is indicative of meningeal irritation and is known as Brudzinski's sign. Lateral inclination of the head may indicate congenital torticollis.
Inspect and palpate the upper extremities. Note the size, color, temperature, and mobility of the joints and abnormalities in the upper extremities. Inspect the palmar creases (Figure 19-2).	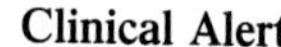 **Clinical Alert** Short, broad extremities, hyperextensible joints, and simian creases may indicate the presence of Down syndrome. The Sydney line is found in children with rubella syndrome.

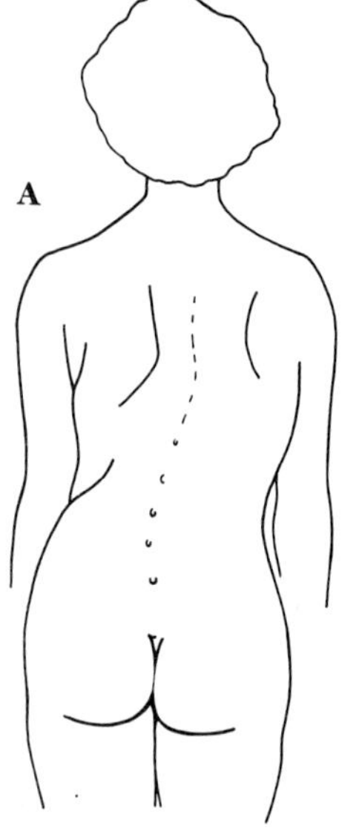

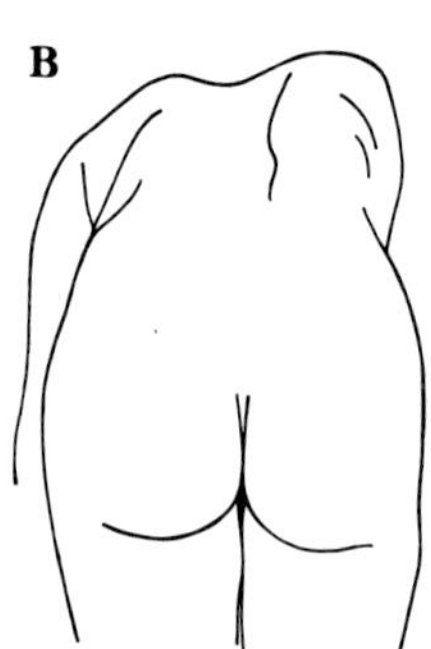

Figure 19-1

Scoliosis. **A,** When child stands, spine assumes lateral curvature and thoracic convexity is present. **B,** When child bends, chest wall on side of convexity is prominent and scapula on side of convexity is elevated.

Assessment	Findings
	Polydactyly (external digits) and syndactyly (webbing) are sometimes found in mentally retarded children.
	Warmth and tenderness of the joints may be indicative of rheumatoid arthritis.
	Widening of the wrist joints may be indicative of rickets.
Assess the strength of the upper extremities by asking the child to squeeze your crossed fingers.	The strength of the upper extremities should be equal. **Clinical Alert** Unilateral weakness may be indicative of hemiparesis or pain.

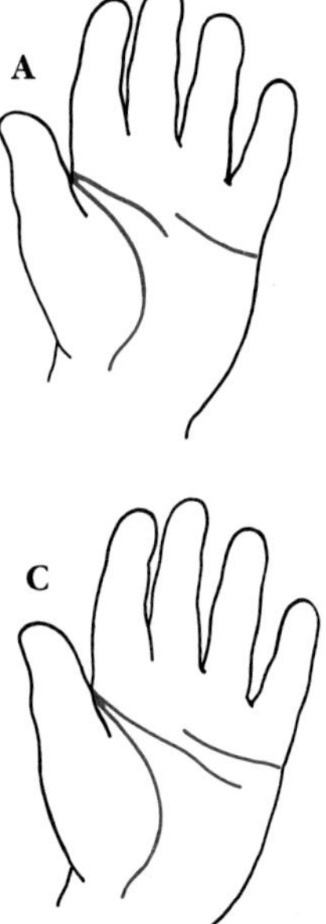

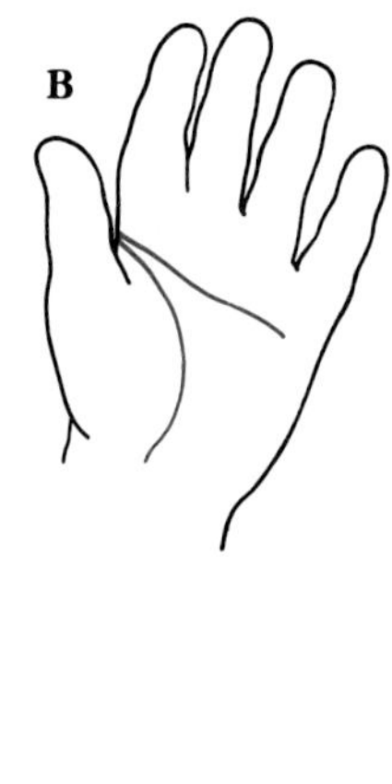

Figure 19-2
Palm creases. A, Normal creases. B, Simian crease. C, Sydney line.

Assessment	Findings
Inspect and palpate the lower extremities. Assess for abnormalities of mobility, length, shape, and pulses.	The feet of infants and toddlers are flat, and the legs are bowed until walking has been firmly established. **Clinical Alert** Fibrosis and contracture of the gluteal and quadriceps muscles occur as complications of intramuscular injections. Observe for limited knee flexion (quadriceps involvement) or hip flexion (gluteal involvement).
Assess for genu varum (bowleg) or genu valgum (knock-knee) by instructing the child to stand with ankles together.	Knock-knee is present until the child is past 7 years of age. **Clinical Alert** In the child older than 2 years of age a space greater than 5 cm (2 in) between the knees is indicative of genu varum. A space greater than 7.5 cm (3 in) between the knees in the child older than 7 years is indicative of genu valgum.
Assess for the presence of clubfoot by lightly scratching the inner and outer soles of the feet. Observe whether the foot assumes a normal angle (i.e., right angle) to the leg when stimulated.	**Clinical Alert** Return of the foot, after stimulation, to a right angle in relation to the leg, may indicate metatarsus varus in an infant with adduction and inversion of the forefoot. Inability of the foot to right itself after stimulation may be indicative of talipes equinovarus (inversion of the forefoot, plantar flexion, and heel inversion) or of talipes calcaneovalgus (eversion of the forefoot and dorsal flexion).

Assessment	Findings
Assess the child for meningeal irritation by flexing the child's hips and then straightening each of the knees (Kernig's sign).	**Clinical Alert** Pain and resistance to straightening of the knees is indicative of meningeal irritation.
Assess for congenital hip dislocation (Table 19-1).	
Assess for strength in the lower limbs by asking the child to push against your hands with the soles of the forefeet.	Strength should be symmetrical in the lower limbs. **Clinical Alert** Unequal strength may indicate hemiparesis or pain.

Related Nursing Diagnoses

Anxiety: Related to pain secondary to injury; surgery; disease.

Comfort, alterations in: Pain related to injury; surgery; disease; position.

Knowledge deficit: Related to care of the child with braces or casts.

Mobility, impaired physical: Secondary to surgery; injury; disease; corrective devices.

Parenting, alterations in: Related to skill deficit; stress.

Self-care deficit: Feeding, bathing/hygiene, dressing secondary to pain; immobility; weakness; corrective devices.

Self-concept: Disturbance in body image, role performance related to limitations in mobility; physical disability.

Table 19-1 Assessment for presence of congenital hip dislocation

Test/Sign	Assessment	Abnormal Findings
Galeazzi's or Allis' sign	Place the infant supine with the hips and knees flexed.	The knees are unequal in height. (Finding may not be apparent in the infant younger than 6 weeks.)
Unequal thigh folds	Place the infant or child prone. Observe symmetry of the thigh folds.	Unequal thigh folds.
Ortolani's sign	Place the infant supine. With your thumbs on the inside of both thighs and your fingertips resting over the trochanter muscles, flex both hips and knees. Abduct each knee until the lateral aspects of the knees touch the examining table. This test is reliable in the neonate and may be performed until the child is 1 year of age. It is less reliable in the older infant.	A click or clunk is heard on abduction.
Barlow's test	Place the infant supine. Flex and slightly adduct both hips while lifting the femur and applying pressure to the trochanter. This test is reliable in the neonate.	Instability of hip joints.
Trendelenburg gait	Observe the gait of the child.	When the child bears weight on the affected side, the unaffected side of the pelvis drops (Figure 19-3).

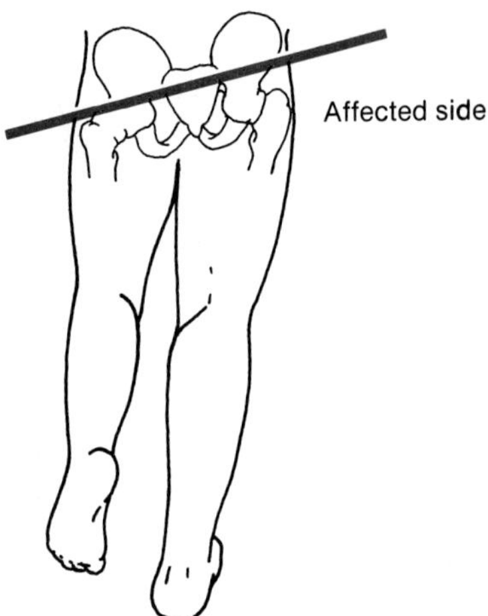

Figure 19-3
Trendelenburg gait.

Nervous System 20

Assessment of the nervous system involves observation and testing of mental status, motor functioning, sensory functioning, cranial nerve functioning, reflexes, and infant automatisms. The thoroughness of assessment depends on the presenting complaint, contributing data from the health assessment, the reason for the assessment, the condition, and the age of the child.

Much of the neurologic assessment can be integrated with other areas of the assessment. Parents can be valuable aides in performing the neurologic assessment of a child because they are more aware of the child's usual functioning. Parental concerns are important in alerting health professionals to delays and impairments.

In performing the neurologic assessment the nurse must be aware of age-appropriate levels of functioning.

Rationale

A thorough neurologic assessment is necessary whenever a child has sustained a fall or has suffered an injury to the head or spine or complains of headaches or has a temperature of unknown origin. Children who have an apparent developmental delay or impairment and those with identified neurologic disorders should also undergo neurologic assessment. Neurologic impairment can delay a child's development and functioning and must be identified early to minimize long-term disability.

Anatomy and Physiology

The nervous system is a complex integrated system, and its scope is beyond that of this text. Essentially the nervous system is composed of the brain, spinal cord, and peripheral nervous system. The brain is divided into the brain stem, the cerebrum, and the cerebellum. Except for the first cranial nerve, the cranial nerves emerge from the brain stem. The brain stem and the spinal cord are continuous. Consciousness arises from interaction between the cerebrum and brain stem. The cerebellum is primarily responsible for coordination. The full number of adult nerve cells is established midway through the prenatal period. Neurons, responsible for memory, consciousness, sensory and motor responses, and thought control, increase in size but not number after birth. Glial cells increase in both size and number until the age of 4 years. Dendrites, responsible for the transmission of impulses across synapses, increase in number and branchings. Axons increase in length. The size of the brain increases from 325 gm (11 oz) at birth to 1000 gm (2.2 lb) by 1 year of age (the adult brain weighs 1400 gm, or approximately 3 lb). Myelinization, begun in the fourth month of gestation, progresses throughout early infancy and childhood, until the child is able to move voluntarily and to engage in higher cortical functions. The order in which myelinization occurs corresponds to the normal sequence of development.

Equipment for Assessment of Nervous System

Two safety pins
Closed jars containing solutions with distinctive odors
Cotton balls
Reflex hammer

Preparation

Ask whether there is a family history of genetic disorders, learning disorders, or birth defects. Inquire whether the mother had difficulties during pregnancy or delivery. Ask the parent about the type of delivery, birth weight of the infant or child, and whether the infant or child had problems after birth. Ask whether the child has or has had recurrent headaches or seizures. If the child has sustained an injury, determine the time of occurrence, the events surrounding the injury, the area of impact, and whether consciousness was lost.

Assessment of Mental Status

Mental status can be assessed informally and formally as the nurse progresses through the examination. Intellectual functioning can be formally assessed through use of the Denver Developmental Screening Test (DDST; *see* Chapter 20), which is administered at specified intervals in some agencies but can be administered any time a problem is suspected. Illness, injury, a strange environment, and the examiner's approach can all influence intellectual functioning, mood, and understanding, so the nurse should compare findings against the parent's observations of the child's behavior.

Assessment	Findings
Observe the child's ability to respond and to follow directions.	**Clinical Alert** A short attention span, easy distractibility, and impulsivity may indicate minimal brain dysfunction.
Observe the infant's or child's response to the mother and to examination. Is the infant or child active, hypoactive, irritable, restless, quiet, cooperative, withdrawn, or belligerent? Can the infant or child withstand momentary delay of gratification? Does the child interrupt or argue?	**Clinical Alert** Hyperactivity (excessive, purposeless movement) or hypoactivity and lability may indicate minimal brain dysfunction.
Assess the child's articulation and fluency of speech.	A child of 3 years should be easily understood.

Assessment of Motor Function

Motor function can be assessed during assessment of the musculoskeletal system.

Assessment	Findings
Observe the infant or child for obvious abnormalities that may influence motor functioning. Specifically, observe the size and shape of the head and inspect the spine for sacs and tufts of hair.	**Clinical Alert** A large head, enlarged frontal area, and tense fontanels (if open) may indicate hydrocephalus. A dimple with a tuft of hair or a sac protruding from the spinal column may indicate spina bifida.
Test muscle strength and symmetry by asking the child to squeeze your fingers, press soles of feet against your hands, and push away pressure exerted on arms and legs.	**Clinical Alert** Report any asymmetry.
Place all joints through range of motion. Note flaccidity or spasticity.	Infants normally have the most flexible range of motion. All school-aged children should be able to perform these activities. **Clinical Alert** Retroflexion of the head, stiffness of the neck, and extension of the extremities accompanies the meningeal irritation of meningitis and intracranial hemorrhage. Head lag after 4 months is an early sign of neurologic damage.
Cerebellar function can be tested by asking the child to hop, skip, or walk heel-to-toe.	**Clinical Alert** Leaning to one side during Romberg's test indicates cerebellar dysfunction.

Assessment	Findings
Romberg's test can be performed by asking the child to stand still, eyes closed and arms at side. Stand near the child to catch the child if leaning occurs.	

Assessment of Sensory Function

Sensory function is assessed during testing of cranial nerve function.

Assessment of Cranial Nerve Function

The function of most of the cranial nerves can be evaluated during other areas of the health assessment (Table 20-1). Particular attention is paid to function of the cranial nerves when neurologic impairment is possible, suspected, or actually present and should be a routine part of assessment in a child with a head injury.

Assessment of the cranial nerves varies with the child's developmental and cognitive levels. Testing of several functions depends on the child's ability to understand and cooperate and therefore such functions cannot be tested in the infant or young child.

Assessment of Deep Tendon Reflexes

Assessment of deep tendon reflexes (Table 20-2) provides information about the intactness of the reflex area. Compare the symmetry and strength of reflexes. Superficial reflexes such as the abdominal reflex, anal reflex, and cremasteric reflex can also be evaluated (Table 20-2), but are usually assessed during other areas of the health assessment. Findings from assessment of deep tendon and superficial reflexes are variable in infancy. Their absence or intensity is not diagnostically significant unless asymmetry is present.

Assessment of Infant Reflexes

Infant reflexes or automatisms (Table 20-3) are particularly useful in assessing the function of the central nervous system. Reflexes should be formally assessed if there is any suggestion of a central nervous disorder. Many reflexes can be assessed during other parts of the health assessment. Knowledge of the reflex aids in education of the parents.

Related Nursing Diagnoses

Bowel elimination, alterations in: Constipation secondary to spinal cord lesions; neurologic disease.

Bowel elimination, alteration in: Incontinence related to ineffective urinary sphincter muscle.

Comfort, alteration in: Pain secondary to increased intracranial pressure.

Communication, impaired verbal: Secondary to deafness; neurologic impairment.

Coping, ineffective family: Compromised related to situational crisis; temporary family disorganization.

Diversional deficit: Related to decreased mobility; difficulty in coordinating movements; physical weakness.

Family processes, altered: Related to situational crisis.

Growth and development, altered: Related to diversional deficit; cerebral impairment.

Injury, high risk for: Related to impaired coordination; immobility.

Mobility, impaired physical: Secondary to neurologic injury; congenital defects.

Parenting, alterations in, potential: Related to skill deficit; knowledge deficit; family stress.

Self-care deficit: Feeding, bathing/hygiene, dressing/grooming, toileting related to muscle weakness; immobility; developmental lag.

Self-concept: Disturbance in body image, self-esteem related to physical limitations; developmental delay; perception of disabilities.

Text continued on p. 217.

Table 20-1 Testing of cranial nerve function

Cranial Nerve	Assessment of Function	Area of Health Assessment into Which Testing Can Be Integrated
I Olfactory	Have the child close eyes and, blocking one nostril at a time; correctly identify distinctive odors (e.g., coffee, oranges).	Head and neck
II Optic*	Check the child's visual acuity, perception of light and color, and peripheral vision. Examine the optic disk.	Eye
III Oculomotor*	Check pupil size and reactivity. Inspect the eyelid for position when open. Have the child follow light or a bright toy through the six cardinal positions of gaze.	Eye
IV Trochlear†	Have the child move eyes downward and inward.	Eye
V Trigeminal*	Palpate the temple and jaw as the child bites down. Assess for symmetry and strength. Determine if the child can detect light touch over the cheeks (a young infant roots when the cheek areas near the mouth are touched). Approaching from the side, touch the colored portion of the eye lightly with a wisp of cotton to test the blink and corneal reflexes.	Eye
VI Abducens†	Ask the child to look sideways. Assess the ability to move eyes laterally.	Eye

VII Facial*	Test the child's ability to identify sweet (sugar), sour (lemon juice), or bitter (quinine) solutions with the anterior tongue. Assess motor function by asking the older child to smile, puff out the cheeks, or show the teeth. (Observe the infant while smiling and crying.)	Head and neck
VIII Acoustic	Test the child's hearing (Chapter 10).	Ear Head and neck
IX Glossopharyngeal†	Test the child's ability to identify the taste of solutions on the posterior tongue.	Head and neck
X Vagus	Assess the child for hoarseness and ability to swallow. Touch a tongue blade to the posterior pharynx to determine if the gag reflex is present (cranial nerves IX and X both participate in this response). *Do not stimulate the gag reflex if there is any suspicion of epiglottitis*. Check that the uvula is in the midline.	Head and neck
XI Accessory†	Have the child attempt to turn the head to the side against resistance. Ask the child to shrug shoulders while downward pressure is applied.	Head and neck
XII Hypoglossal†	Ask the child to stick out the tongue. Inspect the tongue for midline deviation. (Observe the infant's tongue for lateral deviation when crying and laughing.) Listen for the child's ability to pronounce "r" (rabbit, run, Robert). Place a tongue blade against the side of child's tongue and ask the child to move it away. Assess for strength.	Head and neck

*Some portions of function can be assessed in infants and in younger children.
†Only older children can participate in testing.

Table 20-2 Assessment of deep and superficial reflexes

Reflex	Method of Assessment	Usual Finding
Deep Tendon Reflexes		
Biceps	Partially flex the child's forearm. Place your thumb over the antecubital space and strike with the reflex hammer (Figure 20-1, *A*).	Forearm flexes slightly.
Triceps	Bend the child's arm at the elbow while suporting the fore-arm. Strike the triceps tendon above the elbow (Figure 20-1, *B*).	Forearm extends slightly.
Brachioradialis	Place the child's arm and hand in a relaxed position with the palm down. Strike the radius 2.5 cm (1 inch) above the wrist.	Forearm flexes and palm turns upward.
Knee jerk or patellar	Have the child sit on a table or on the parent's lap with legs flexed and dangling. Strike the patellar tendon just below the kneecap.	Lower leg extends.

Achilles	Have the child sit on a table or on the parent's lap with legs flexed and support the foot lightly. Strike the Achilles tendon.	Foot plantar flexes (points downward). Rapid, rhythmic plantar flexion of the foot may occur in newborn infants (up to 10 flexions may be noted).
Superficial Reflexes		
Abdominal	Stroke the skin toward the umbilicus. Assess the reflex in all four quadrants. The abdominal reflex may not be present for the first 6 months. (Can be incorporated into assessment of the abdomen.)	Umbilicus moves toward the stimulus.
Cremasteric	Stroke the upper inner thigh. (Can be integrated into assessment of the abdominal or genital area.)	Testes retract into the inguinal canal.
Anal	Stimulate the skin in the perianal area. (Can be incorporated into assessment of the rectal area.)	Brisk contraction of the anal sphincter occurs.

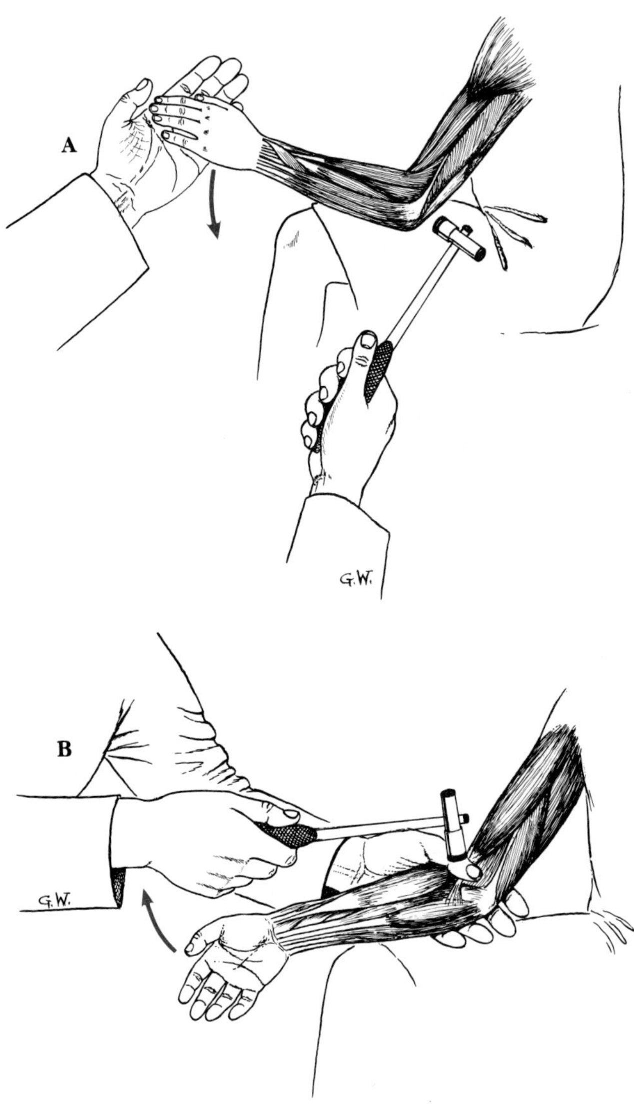

Figure 20-1
Assessment of deep tendon reflexes. A, Biceps. B, Triceps.
From Whaley LF, Wong DL: Nursing care of infants and children, ed 4, St Louis, 1991, Mosby–Year Book.

Table 20-3 Infant reflexes (automatisms)

Reflex	Description	Method of Assessment	Significance of Findings
Blinking (dazzle)	Closes eyelids in response to bright light. Present during first year of life.	Shine light into infant's eyes.	Absence of reflex suggests blindness.
Babinski's sign	Toes fan and big toe dorsiflexes. Present until 2 years of age.	Stroke sole of foot along outer edge, beginning from heel.	Fanning of toes and dorsiflexion of great toe after 2 years of age suggests lesion in extrapyramidal tract.
Crawling	Infant makes crawling movements with arms and legs when placed on abdomen.	Place infant prone on flat surface.	Asymmetry of movements suggests neurologic disorder.
Dance or stepping	Infant's feet move up and down when feet lightly touch firm surface. Present for first 4-8 weeks.	Hold infant so that feet lightly touch firm surface.	Persistence of reflex beyond 4-8 weeks is abnormal.
Extrusion	Tongue extends outward when touched. Present until 4 months of age.	Touch tongue with tip of tongue blade.	Persistent extension of tongue may indicate Down's syndrome.

Continued.

Table 20-3 Infant reflexes (automatisms)—cont'd

Reflex	Description	Method of Assessment	Significance of Findings
Galant's (trunk incurvation)	Back moves toward side that is stimulated. Present for first 4-8 weeks.	Stroke infant's back along side of spine from shoulder to buttocks.	Absence of reflex may indicate transverse spinal cord lesions.
Moro's	Arms extend, fingers fan, head is thrown back, and legs may flex weakly. Arms return to center with hands clasped. Spine and lower extremities extend. Strongest during first 2 months. Disappears at 3-4 months.	Change infant's position abruptly or jar table.	Persistence of reflex beyond 4 months is suggestive of brain damage. Persistence beyond 6 months is highly indicative of brain damage. Asymmetry of responses is indicative of hemiparesis, fracture of clavicle, or injury to brachial plexus. Absence of response in lower extremities is indicative of congenital hip dislocation or low spinal cord injury.

Neck righting	When infant is supine, shoulder and trunk and then pelvis turn toward direction in which infant is turned. Persists for first 10 months.	Place infant supine. Attempt to attract infant's attention to one side.	Absence or persistence beyond 10 months suggests central nervous system disorders.
Palmar grasp	Infant's fingers curve around finger placed in infant's palm from ulnar side. Palmar grasp disappears by 3-4 months.	Place finger into infant's palm from ulnar side. If reflex is weak or absent offer infant bottle or soother as sucking enhances reflex.	Asymmetric flexion is indicative of paralysis. Persistence of grasp reflex is indicative of cerebral disorder.
Rooting	Infant turns in direction that cheek is stroked. Reflex disappears at 3-4 months, but may persist for up to 12 months, especially during sleep.	Stroke corners of infant's mouth or midline of lips.	Absence of reflex is indicative of severe neurologic disorder.
Startle	Infant extends and flexes arms in response to loud noise. Hands remain clenched. Reflex disappears after 4 months of age.	Clap hands loudly.	Absence of reflex is indicative of hearing impairment.

Continued.

Table 20-3 Infant reflexes (automatisms)—cont'd

Reflex	Description	Method of Assessment	Significance of Findings
Sucking	Infant sucks strongly in response to stimulation. Reflex persists during infancy and may occur during sleep without stimulation.	Offer infant bottle or soother.	Weak or absent reflex suggests developmental delay or neurologic abnormality.
Tonic neck	Infant assumes fencing position when head is turned to one side. Arm and leg extend on side to which head is turned and flex on opposite side. Normally reflex should not occur each time head is turned. Appears at approximately 2 months, disappears at 6 months.	Turn head quickly to one side.	It is considered abnormal if response occurs each time head is turned. Persistence is indicative of major cerebral damage.

Skin integrity, impaired: Actual or high risk for related to immobility; urinary incontinence; fecal incontinence.

Social isolation: Related to impaired mobility; disturbance in self concept.

Thought processes, altered: Secondary to cerebral dysfunction.

Urinary elimination, alteration in patterns of: Related to ineffective urinary sphincter muscle.

PART

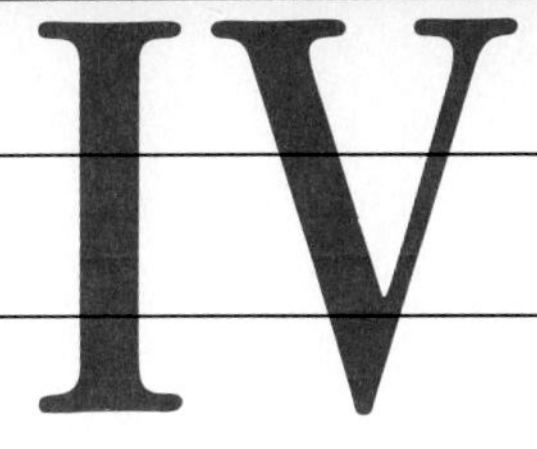

GENERAL ASSESSMENT

Development 21

Development is multifactorial and is the interplay among temperament, environment, and biophysical factors. Many observations about development can be made informally during the health interview and the neurologic and musculoskeletal assessments. However, some observations need to be made more formally using tools such as the Denver Developmental Screening Test (DDST) and other objective tests.

The nurse needs to be aware that *normal encompasses a wide range of behavior at any given stage* and that delays in development can rarely be attributed to only one factor. Knowledge of behaviors that can be expected at various stages is essential to assessment of development.

Rationale

Complete periodic, systematic assessment of development enables early detection of problems, identification of parental and child concerns, anticipatory guidance, and teaching about age-appropriate expected behaviors. Judgments about an infant's or child's development must *never* rest solely on one assessment of development. Illness, stress, the examiner's approach, and a strange environment can alter a child's usual performance.

Preparation

Ask the parent to describe the infant's or child's development. Inquire whether the parent has specific concerns about the infant's or child's development. Ask about the mother's prenatal history, including miscarriages, stillbirths, exposure to medications or radiation, drug or alcohol use, maternal endocrine disorders, toxemia, hydramnios, infection, or abnormal bleeding. Inquire about the birth history of the infant or child, including type of delivery, fetal distress, birth weight, prematurity, respiratory problems, jaundice, hypoglycemia, seizures, irritability, poor muscle tone, or feeding problems.

Assessment of Development Using Denver Developmental Screening Tests

The Denver Developmental Screening Test (DDST) and Denver Developmental Screening Test Revised (DDST-R) are *not* IQ tests, but standard developmental tools that can be used for children from birth to 6 years to *screen* for developmental delays and to monitor children who are at risk for developmental delays. The tests do not tell *why* developmental delays have occurred.

Equipment for Assessment with DDST

Approved DDST kit

Method of Assessment

1. Draw a line from top to bottom of the DDST or DDST-R score sheet (Appendix A) in the appropriate age slot.
2. Test all items that intersect the vertical line. If a number appears on an item, refer to the back of the sheet for specific instructions regarding testing.
3. Mark "F" on items that have been failed, "P" on items that have been passed, and "R" on items that were refused.

Significance of Findings

The average child is not expected to pass all test items. A test item that is failed is not of concern unless it is located to the immediate *left* of the vertical age line, which means that 90% of children younger than the child can perform the task. This is considered a developmental delay. A child is not considered developmentally delayed unless all items intersecting the vertical age line have been administered and there are at least three failures in each category. If a child does not perform well during testing or refuses to perform, a second screening should be carried out at a later date.

Assessment of Growth and Development

Assessment of development requires knowledge of what can be expected at various stages in development. Table 21-1 gives a

Text continued on p. 245.

Table 21-1 Summary of normal growth and development

Age	Physical/Motor	Language	Cognition	Socialization
1 month	Average weekly weight gain 140-200 gm (5-6 oz) until 6 months of age. Average monthly gain in length 2.5 cm (1 in) until 6 months of age. Obligate nose breather. Head sags when not supported. Back rounded in sitting position. Hands held in fists. Can turn head to side when prone. Makes crawling movements when prone.	Cries when uncomfortable. Makes low throaty sounds.	SENSORIMOTOR PHASE *Reflective stage* Egocentric No intentionality; no expectations.	Regards faces intently.

Continued.

Table 21-1 Summary of normal growth and development—cont'd

Age	Physical/Motor	Language	Cognition	Socialization
2 months	Posterior fontanel closes. Can lift head 45° when prone. When supported in sitting position, head is held up but bobs forward. Visually pursues objects and sounds. Hands held open more. Grasp reflex fading.	Crying differentiated. Coos. Vocalizes.	*Primary circular reactions stage.* Responds differently to different objects. Voluntarily repeats activities, thereby demonstrating beginning connection between action and result. Anticipates feeding. Begins to separate self from others.	May smile socially.
3 months	Holds hands in front and stares at them. Holds rattle but does not	Squeals. Laughs. Vocalizes in	As for 2 months.	Recognizes familiar face and unfamil-

	reach for it. Raises chest, supported on forearms. Little head lag. Visually pursues sound by turning head. Able to bear some weight on legs when held in standing position. Palmar grasp reflex weakening.	response to other voices.		iar situations. Stops crying when parent approaches.
4 months	Holds head steady in sitting position. Almost no head lag when pulled to sitting position. Sits erect if propped. Lifts head and shoulders 90° when prone. Turns from back to side. Plays with hands. Reaches for objects but overshoots.	Makes consonant sounds (b, g, k, n, p) interspersed with vowel-like sounds. Vocalization varies with mood.	As for 2 months.	Sociable. Bored if left alone. Demands attention by fussing.

Continued.

Table 21-1 Summary of normal growth and development—cont'd

Age	Physical/Motor	Language	Cognition	Socialization
4 months—cont'd	Grasps objects with both hands. Visually pursues objects that have been dropped. Begins drooling. Moro, tonic neck, extrusion, and rooting reflexes disappear. Sleeps 10-12 hours at night. Naps 2-3 times a day.			
5 months	No head lag. Back straight when pulled to sitting. Bears most of weight on legs when standing. Sits for longer periods if back supported. Plays with feet. Takes objects to mouth at will.	As for 4 months.	*Secondary circular reactions stage.* Searches for objects at point of disappearance. Recognizes partially hidden objects. Repeats interesting actions.	Recognizes strangers. May have rapid mood swings. Vocalizes displeasure if preferred object is taken.

	Teeth may begin to erupt.		Wide repertoire of activities (kicking, batting, pulling, patting) that produce novel results. Imitates others.	
6 months	Average weekly gain 90-150 gm (3-5 oz) for next 6 months. Chews and bites. May hold own bottle but prefers it to be held. Lifts chest and abdomen off flat surface, bearing weight on hands. Sits in highchair with back straight. Can turn completely from stomach to back to stomach. Picks up objects that have been dropped.	Vocalizes to mirror. Makes one-syllable sounds (ma, da, uh). Begins to mimic sounds (e.g., coughing).	As for 5 months.	Shows fear of strangers. Holds out arms when wants to be picked up. Becomes excited when familiar persons approach. Laughs when head covered with towel.

Continued.

Table 21-1 Summary of normal growth and development—cont'd

Age	Physical/Motor	Language	Cognition	Socialization
6 months—cont'd	Manipulates small objects. Pulls feet to mouth. Adjusts posture to visually pursue an object. Exhibits Landau reflex (when held prone, head raises and spine and legs extend).			
7 months	Sits in tripod position. Lifts head off table if supine. Bounces if held in standing position. Transfers cube from hand to hand. Holds cube in each hand. Bangs cube on table. Rakes at small objects. Can approach toy and grasp it with one hand.	Chains syllables (mama, dada) but does not attach meaning. Is able to produce four distinct vowel sounds.	As for 5 months.	Increasing fear of strangers. Imitative. Coughs, snorts to attract attention. Closes lips in response to dislike of food. Bites and mouths.

	Responds to own name. Evidences taste preferences.			Plays Peek-a-boo.
8 months	Sits alone steadily. May stand holding onto something. Beginning pincer (thumb-finger) grasp. Regards a third cube while holding a cube in each hand. Releases objects voluntarily. Rings bell purposely. Reaches for toys out of reach. May have night awakenings. Patterns emerge in bowel and bladder elimination.	Makes d, t, w sounds. Responds to simple commands.	As for 5 months. Coordination of secondary schemes. Object permanence.	Increased stranger anxiety and fear of separation from parent. Begins to respond to "no-no." Searches for hidden objects. Shows interest in pleasing parent.
9 months	Pulls self to standing position. Crawls, perhaps backward, at first.		Beginning of intelligence. Assigns symbols to events.	May show fear of going to bed or of being alone.

Continued.

Table 21-1 Summary of normal growth and development—cont'd

Age	Physical/Motor	Language	Cognition	Socialization
9 months—cont'd	Recovers sitting position if leaning forward, but cannot do so if leaning sideways.		Goal-directed activities.	
10 months	Crawls, pulling self forward by hands. Stands holding onto furniture. May cruise (step sideways holding onto furniture). Recovers balance readily if sitting.	Comprehends dada, mama. May say one word.	As for 9 months.	Waves bye-bye. Extends toys to others but does not release toy. Repeats activities that attract attention. Plays pat-a-cake. Cries when scolded.
11 months	Creeps with abdomen off floor.	Imitates speech sounds.	As for 9 months.	Expresses frustration when

	Pivots when sitting (reaches backward to pick up an object). Intentionally drops objects for them to be picked up. Places objects inside each other. Holds crayon to make mark on paper.			restricted. Plays so-big, up-down, peek-a-boo.
12 months	Birth weight tripled. Head and chest circumference equal. Cruises well. Walks with help. Can sit from standing without help. Drinks from cup and eats from spoon but requires help. Cooperates in dressing. Neat pincer grasp. Turns several pages of book at a time.	Says two or more words in addition to mama and dada. Recognizes objects by name. Imitates sounds of animals.	As for 9 months.	Responds to simple commands. Explores actively. Clings to mother in unfamiliar situations. May take security objects. Shows emotions.

Continued.

Table 21-1 Summary of normal growth and development—cont'd

Age	Physical/Motor	Language	Cognition	Socialization
12 months—cont'd	Lumbar nerve develops, with resulting lordosis when walking.			
13-18 months	Anterior fontanel closes. Abdomen protrudes. Walks with wide-based gait. Walks upstairs with help, creeps downstairs. Throws ball overhand. Seats self on small chair. Climbs. Pulls toys behind and pushes light furniture. Imitates housework. Puts shaped objects into holes. Scribbles vigorously. Imitates vertical and circular strokes.	By 15 months, infant able to say four to six words, and by 18 months 10 words or more. Points to desired object. Points to two or three body parts (18 months).	*Tertiary circular reactions stage*. Trial and error learning. Active experimentation. Solicits help of adults to bring about results. Understands relationship between object and use.	Drinks well from cup but may drop it when finished. Holds cup well in both hands. Uses spoon but turns bowl of spoon downward before it reaches mouth. May discard bottle. Less fearful of strangers.

	Builds tower of two or three cubes. Sleeps 10-12 hours. Has one afternoon nap. May uncover self during sleep.			Hugs and kisses significant others and pictures in a book. Temper tantrums begin. Beginning sense of ownership. Takes off simple clothes.
24 months	Average yearly weight gain 1.8-2.7 kg (4-6 lb). Chest circumference larger than head circumference. Physiologic systems stable except for reproductive and endocrine systems. Gait steadier, more adult. Jumps crudely. May pedal tricycle. Walks up and down stairs	Approximately 300 words in vocabulary. Short sentences of two or three words. Uses pronouns. Gives first name. Verbalizes need for food,	Inventions of new means through mental combinations. Beginning of mental problem solving and play. Has insight, foresight, forethought. Able to delay imitation	Dawdles. Negativistic. Temper tantrums decrease. Treats other children as objects. Wants to make friends but doesn't

Continued.

Table 21-1 Summary of normal growth and development—cont'd

Age	Physical/Motor	Language	Cognition	Socialization
24 months—cont'd	with two feet on each step. Holds onto rail. Picks up objects without falling. Kicks ball forward without overbalancing. Turns doorknob and unscrews lids. Builds tower of six or seven cubes. Turns pages of book one at a time. May be daytime toilet trained.	drink, and toilet.	for several days.	know how. Cannot share possessions. Engages in parallel play. Shows increased independence from mother. Chews with mouth closed. Uses straw. Puts on simple clothing.
30 months	Birth weight quadrupled. Primary dentition complete. Builds tower of eight cubes. Copies circle from model. Throws large ball 1.2-1.5 m (4-5 ft).	Gives first and last names. Enjoys rhymes and singing.	PREOPERATIONAL PHASE *Preconceptual stage* Symbols increas-	Separates easily from parent. Notices sex difference. Independent in toileting ex-

	Takes a few steps on tiptoe.		ingly used. Egocentric. Representative thought. Symbolic and fantasy play. Beginning to understand concept of time.	cept for wiping.
36 months	Average yearly weight gain 1.8-2.7 kg (4-6 lb). Balances on one foot for 5 seconds. Jumps from a low step. Walks upstairs, alternating feet. May attempt to dance but balance still insecure. Pours fluid well from a pitcher. Begins to use scissors. Strings large beads.	Vocabulary of about 900 words. Talks in sentences of about six words. Uses telegraphic speech. Asks many questions.	Repeats three numbers. Remainder as for 30 months.	Less negativistic. Friendly. Begins to understand taking turns. Able to share but uses "mine" often. Begins to learn meaning of simple rules, but rules sub-

Continued.

Table 21-1 Summary of normal growth and development—cont'd

Age	Physical/Motor	Language	Cognition	Socialization
36 months—cont'd	Builds tower of 9 or 10 cubes. Copies cross (X) from model. Washes hands. May be nighttime toilet trained. Sleeps 10-15 hours. Takes fewer naps.			ject to own interpretation. Names appropriate sex of other. Boys tend to identify more strongly with father. May dress with minimal assistance. Feeds self completely. Begins to use fork but holds it in fist. Uses adult form of chewing. May have fears,

				especially of dark or animals.
48 months	Length at birth doubled. Balances on one foot for 10 seconds. Hops on one foot. Catches bounced ball. Laces shoes. Imitates bridge with cubes. Uses scissors to cut out picture. Immunoglobulin G reaches adult levels. Draws man in three parts.	Vocabulary of 1500 words. Knows simple songs. Exaggerates, boasts, may be mildly profane. Understands concepts of under, on top of, beside, in front of. Understands simple analogies.	*Intuitive stage* Time linked with daily events. Counts but does not clearly understand what numbers mean. Believes thoughts cause events. Cannot conserve matter. Egocentricism decreases. Repeats four numbers. Names one or more coins.	Tattles. May have imaginary playmate. Independent. Aggressive. Takes out aggression on family members. Exhibits mood swings. Engages in cooperative group play. Enjoys entertaining. Do's and don'ts important.

Continued.

Table 21-1 Summary of normal growth and development—cont'd

Age	Physical/Motor	Language	Cognition	Socialization
48 months—cont'd				Identifies with parent of opposite sex.
5 years	Permanent dentition may begin. Handedness established. Jumps rope. Walks backward heel-to-toe. May be able to tie shoelaces. Can form some letters correctly. May print first name. Draws man in six or seven parts. Uses scissors or pencil well. Copies triangle and diamond.	Vocabulary of about 2100 words. Talks constantly. Asks meanings of words.	Uses time words with more comprehension. Interested in facts associated with environment. Names four or more colors. Names coins. Names days of week.	Comfortable. Trustworthy. Fewer fears. Eager to do things the right way. May seek out mother more often because of more outside activities such as school. Identifies strongly with

				parent of same sex.
6 years	Dexterity increasing. Jumps rope. Skates, rides bicycle. May sew crudely.	Describes objects in pictures.	Knows right from left. Recognizes many shapes. Reads from memory. Obeys three commands in succession.	Enjoys bossing others. May be defiant and rude. Jealousy of younger siblings more apparent. May have temper tantrums. Cheats to win. Enjoys table games.
7 years		Mechanical in reading. May skip words such as he, it.	Repeats three numbers backward. Reads time to quarter hour.	Enjoys teasing. Girls play with girls, and boys with boys. Modest about sexual matters.

Continued.

Table 21-1 Summary of normal growth and development—cont'd

Age	Physical/Motor	Language	Cognition	Socialization
7 years—cont'd				Anxious over failures. Occasional periods of shyness or sadness. Increasing interest in spiritual matters.
8-9 years	Increased speed and smoothness in motor activities. Uses common tools such as hammer and household utensils. More individual variation in skills.		*Concrete operational stage (7-11 years)* Age of relational thinking. Able to classify, seriate, arrange in hierarchies. Learns principle of conservation. Knows date.	Expansive. Wants to become involved in everything. Actively seeks company of others. Likes clubs and fads. Hero worship

			Gives days of week and months in order. Counts backward from 20 to 1. Makes change correctly from a quarter.	begins. Likes to help. May reject Santa Claus, Easter Bunny. May show lack of interest in God.
10-12 years	Slow increase in height. Rapid increase in weight. Body changes associated with puberty may appear. Remainder of teeth erupt. Cooks, sews, paints, draws. Washes and dries own hair.	Likes writing letters. Reads for enjoyment or practical purposes.	*FORMAL OPERATIONAL PHASE* Logical thinking and ability to use abstract thought develops. Thinking is reflective, futuristic, multidimensional.	Very interested in reading, science, creative endeavors. Demonstrative. Peers and parents important. Conversational. Beginning interest in opposite sex.

Continued.

Table 21-1 Summary of normal growth and development—cont'd

Age	Physical/Motor	Language	Cognition	Socialization
Early adolescence	Maximum increase in height, weight. Girls may commence menses. Girls may look more obese. May be clumsy and have poor posture. May have fatigue. Immunoglobulins A and M reach adult levels.	Spends long periods on telephone.	Clumsy and inconsistent in abstract thinking. Low point in creativity.	Differences intolerable. Conforms to group standards. Tries on various roles. Ambivalent. Mood-swings. Period of intense conflict with parents. Boys gravitate toward sports. Girls discuss clothes, makeup. Daydreams a great deal.

Middle adolescence	Girls reach physical maturity.	Able to maintain an argument.	Increased capacity for abstract reasoning. Enjoys intellectual powers. Concerned with philosophic and social problems. Creative period.	Introspective. Emotions still labile. Parent-child relationship may reach low point. Disengagement from dependent parent-child relationship occurs. Fears rejection by peers. Adheres to group norms. Sexual preference becoming established. Dating becomes important.

Continued.

Table 21-1 Summary of normal growth and development—cont'd

Age	Physical/Motor	Language	Cognition	Socialization
Late adolescence	Boys reach physical maturity.		Complex thinking. Creativity fading.	Pursues career. Sexual identity established. More comfortable with self. Fewer conflicts with family. Peer group less important. Emotions more controlled. Forms stable relationships.

general summary of normal growth and development that can be used during observation of an infant or child.

Related Nursing Diagnoses

Anxiety: Related to separation from parents; peer relationships; achievement; sexual development; independence; parenting.

Coping, ineffective individual: Related to poor self-esteem; developmental tasks; physical and emotional changes; increasing independence from family; peer relationships; heterosexual relationships; sexual awareness; career choices; leaving home.

Coping, ineffective family: Related to lack of knowledge about normal child development; adolescent rebellion.

Grieving, situational: Related to changes in life-style; child leaving home.

Injury, high risk for: Related to home environmental hazards; use of bicycles, automobiles; use of drugs, alcohol; increasing independence in activities.

Knowledge deficit: Related to growth and development of the infant or child; contraception.

Parenting, alteration in: Related to needs precipitated by growth and development of the infant or child.

Sexuality patterns, altered: Related to the physical and emotional changes of adolescence.

Assessment of Child Abuse

22

Rationale

Although the exact number of cases of child abuse and neglect is difficult to determine because of difficulties in identification and reporting, estimates place the incidence in the United States from 200,000 to 4 million cases annually. Minimally, 4,000 children die annually of abuse and neglect. The preeminence of abuse and neglect necessitates that nurses be alert to specific maltreatment indicators when assessing children.

Development of Abuse

Child abuse, defined as physical, psychological, sexual, or social injury damage, maltreatment, or corruption of a child, can be traced to parents, siblings, relatives, friends, professionals, and others who encounter the child. Neglect usually refers to intentional or unintentional failure to supply a child with the basic necessities of life.

Familial violence/abuse is generally considered to be the way in which a family system expresses its dysfunction. These families, which demonstrate a number of characteristics (see Table 22-1), may be geographically and emotionally isolated and may tend to discount, deny, or be unaware of the seriousness of their problems. A number of factors (see box on p. 248) can place a family at risk for violence and abuse, and awareness of these factors can assist the nurse in assessing families at all stages in family development.

Table 22-1 Characteristics of abusive and violent families

Characteristic	Manifestations
Boundary	Rigid and inflexible. Little contact with outside social support systems. Within the family, there may be blurring of generational boundaries so that a daughter, for example, takes on the role of adult female sexual partner. Parent may seek gratification from child.
Affective tone	Helplessness, crisis, anger, powerlessness, depression. Competition for caring. Little empathy or evidence of nurturance, caring.
Control	Caring confused with conflict and abuse. Imbalance in power, often male or adult dominated. Members facilitate victim roles.
Instrumental functioning	Confusion about roles. Adult and child roles may be reversed. Intense attention to tasks or ineffective performance of tasks. Inappropriate age-related expectations of children.
Communication	Poor; double messages; mixed messages. Threats, sarcasm, blaming, demeaning communication. Incongruence in communication. Lack of meaningful communication. Family secrets common.
Role stereotyping	Traditionalist. Rigid. Role confusion, blurring, and reversal. Parental coalition limited or absent.

Factors that Place Families At Risk for Child Abuse and Neglect

- History of childhood abuse, neglect, deprivation in parent(s)
- Decreased knowledge of parenting skills and normal child development
- Marital discord
- Interspousal violence
- Parental separation
- Chronically ill parent(s)
- Parental substance abuse
- Diminished self-esteem in parent(s)
- Blended family
- Teenage parents
- Prematurity of infant(s)
- Developmental delays in child(ren)
- Social isolation
- Illegitimacy

Assessment of Abuse/Neglect in Children

Assessment of abuse and neglect should be ongoing and an integral part of a total health assessment. Findings that indicate abuse (see box on pp 249-250) must be clearly documented and reported. Care must be taken to describe, not interpret, behaviors and communications. If a child indicates that abuse has occurred, the child's report must be accepted and the child must be shown acceptance. Further exploration of abuse in the younger child can be facilitated by trained professionals through play, particularly through drawings and dramatic activities.

Indicators of Abuse and Neglect in Children

Emotional Abuse and Neglect

Failure to thrive (feeding difficulties, abnormally low height and weight, hypotonia, delayed dentition, developmental delays, passivity, self-stimulation behaviors)
Feeding disorders (rumination, anorexia)
Speech disorders
Enuresis
Sleep disorders
Psychosomatic complaints (headaches, nausea, abdominal pain)
Self-stimulation behaviors (rocking, head-banging, sucking)
Lack of stranger anxiety (infancy)
Withdrawal, indifference
Inhibition of play
Antisocial behavior (stealing, cruelty, destructiveness)
Suicide attempts

Physical Abuse and Neglect

Bruises and welts (on soft tissue areas such as buttocks, mouth, thighs, or torso; may be in various stages of healing)
Burns (may be friction, immersion, or pattern burns; located on soles of feet, palms of hands, buttocks, back)
Fractures (multiple; various stages of healing; spiral fractures; fractures of skull, face, nose, and long bones more common)
Lacerations and abrasions (especially found on backs of arms, legs, torso, external genitalia, face, mouth, lips, or gums; human bite marks may be evident)
Whiplash
Chemical injuries (unexplained poisoning or illness)
Failure to thrive
Signs of malnutrition (thinness, abdominal distention)
Unattended needs (glasses, dental work, physical injuries)
Poor physical hygiene (severe diaper rash, dirty hair, persistent body odor)

Continued.

Indicators of Abuse and Neglect in Children—cont'd

Physical Abuse and Neglect—cont'd

Unclean or inappropriate dress
Frequent accidents due to neglect
Unusual wariness or fear of adults
Withdrawal and/or lack of reaction
Inappropriate displays of friendliness and affection
Acting out (hitting, punching, biting, vandalism or shoplifting)
Absenteeism from school
Arriving early at school and staying late
Dullness, lethargy, inactivity
Begging and stealing food
Consistent lack of supervision

Sexual Abuse

Bruises, bleeding, or lacerations of external genitalia, vagina, or anus
Bloody or stained underwear
Difficulty walking and/or sitting
Venereal disease in young child
Vaginal or penile discharge
Recurrent vaginal infections
Pain on urination
Persistent sore throats of unknown origin
Pregnancy in adolescent females
Withdrawal
Preoccupation with fantasies
Unusual or precocious sexual behavior and knowledge
Sudden changes in behavior (nightmares, fears, phobias, regression, acute anxiety)
Noticeable personality changes
Anger at mother (in incestuous relationships)
Poor peer relationships
Infantile behaviors
Self-mutilation
Suicidal thoughts or attempts
Abuse of drugs or alcohol

Related Nursing Diagnoses

Activity intolerance: Related to fatigue; inadequate intake of protein and calories.

Communication, impaired: Verbal related to fear, dysfunctional family relationships, social isolation, denial.

Coping, ineffective family: Related to family history of sexual abuse, multiple stressors, maturity of parents, childhood abuse or neglect of parents.

Family process, alteration in: Related to dysfunctional communication.

Fear: Related to knowledge deficit, dysfunctional family relationships.

Growth and development, alterations in: Related to deficit of protein and calories; neglect; lack of emotional caring; decreased stimulation.

Health maintenance, alterations in: Related to lack of knowledge; abuse; neglect.

Infection: Related to inappropriate sexual contact, injury.

Knowledge deficit: Related to normal development.

Mobility, impaired physical: Secondary to abuse, neglect.

Nutrition, alterations in: Less than body requirements related to lack of knowledge of adequate nutrition; neglect; physical injury to face or abdomen.

Self-concept: Disturbances in body image, self-esteem, role performance, personal identity related to dysfunctional family relationships; physical or sexual abuse.

Sexuality patterns, altered: Related to abuse.

Skin integrity, impairment of: Related to neglect; physical or sexual abuse.

PART

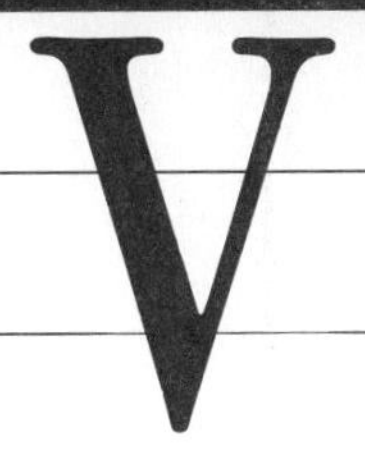

CONCLUDING THE ASSESSMENT

23 Completing the Examination

- Signal to the child and the parent that the assessment is at an end.
- Provide an opportunity for the parent and child to ask questions or verbalize concerns.
- Assist the child to dress.
- Praise the child for cooperation during the examination. Offer reassurance and empathy to the child who has been frightened or upset.
- Express appreciation to the parent for assistance.
- Share assessment findings with the parent (and child, if appropriate). *If findings are abnormal, the beginning practitioner should confirm them with a more experienced nurse before sharing with the parents and child.*
- Findings that initiate concern for the *immediate welfare* of the child, such as respiratory difficulties and abnormal neurologic signs, should be *communicated directly and quickly* to the physician and appropriate health care givers.
- Findings should be organized and written down as soon as possible after assessment to avoid inaccurate or vague documentation of detail (see Appendix E).
- If unsure of the correct terminology, describe the findings.
- Avoid use of "good" and "normal." These terms are subjective and vary greatly from nurse to nurse. Use specific, descriptive terms. Measurements, where possible, should be included.
- Findings should be documented in a way that is organized, concise, specific, accurate, complete, confidential, and legible.

APPENDICES

Appendix A Developmental Assessment

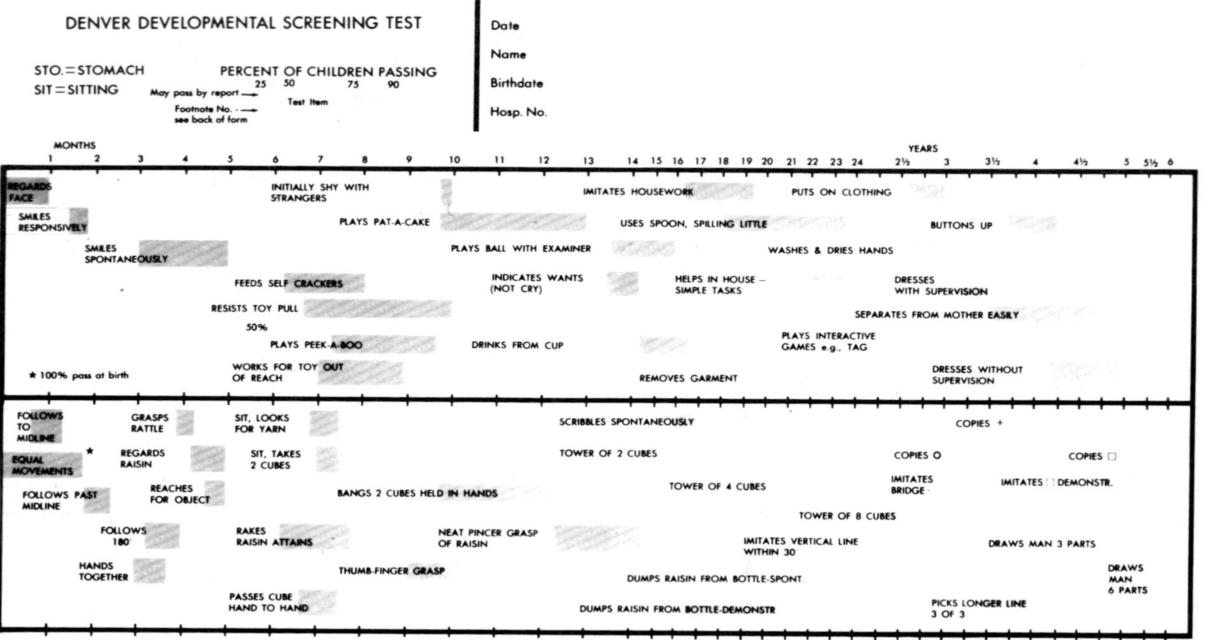

DENVER DEVELOPMENTAL SCREENING TEST

STO. = STOMACH
SIT = SITTING

PERCENT OF CHILDREN PASSING
25 50 75 90
May pass by report
Footnote No. - see back of form
Test Item

Date
Name
Birthdate
Hosp. No.

MONTHS
1 2 3 4 5 6 7 8 9 10 11 12 13 14 15 16 17 18 19 20 21 22 23 24
YEARS
2½ 3 3½ 4 4½ 5 5½ 6

PERSONAL - SOCIAL

REGARDS FACE
SMILES RESPONSIVELY
SMILES SPONTANEOUSLY
INITIALLY SHY WITH STRANGERS
PLAYS PAT-A-CAKE
FEEDS SELF CRACKERS
RESISTS TOY PULL
50%
PLAYS PEEK-A-BOO
WORKS FOR TOY OUT OF REACH
★ 100% pass at birth
PLAYS BALL WITH EXAMINER
INDICATES WANTS (NOT CRY)
DRINKS FROM CUP
IMITATES HOUSEWORK
USES SPOON, SPILLING LITTLE
HELPS IN HOUSE – SIMPLE TASKS
REMOVES GARMENT
PUTS ON CLOTHING
WASHES & DRIES HANDS
PLAYS INTERACTIVE GAMES e.g., TAG
DRESSES WITH SUPERVISION
SEPARATES FROM MOTHER EASILY
BUTTONS UP
DRESSES WITHOUT SUPERVISION

FINE MOTOR-ADAPTIVE

FOLLOWS TO MIDLINE
EQUAL MOVEMENTS ★
FOLLOWS PAST MIDLINE
FOLLOWS 180°
HANDS TOGETHER
GRASPS RATTLE
REGARDS RAISIN
REACHES FOR OBJECT
SIT, LOOKS FOR YARN
SIT, TAKES 2 CUBES
RAKES RAISIN ATTAINS
PASSES CUBE HAND TO HAND
BANGS 2 CUBES HELD IN HANDS
THUMB-FINGER GRASP
NEAT PINCER GRASP OF RAISIN
SCRIBBLES SPONTANEOUSLY
TOWER OF 2 CUBES
TOWER OF 4 CUBES
DUMPS RAISIN FROM BOTTLE-SPONT.
DUMPS RAISIN FROM BOTTLE-DEMONSTR
IMITATES VERTICAL LINE WITHIN 30°
TOWER OF 8 CUBES
COPIES O
IMITATES BRIDGE
PICKS LONGER LINE 3 OF 3
COPIES +
IMITATES □ DEMONSTR.
DRAWS MAN 3 PARTS
COPIES □
DRAWS MAN 6 PARTS

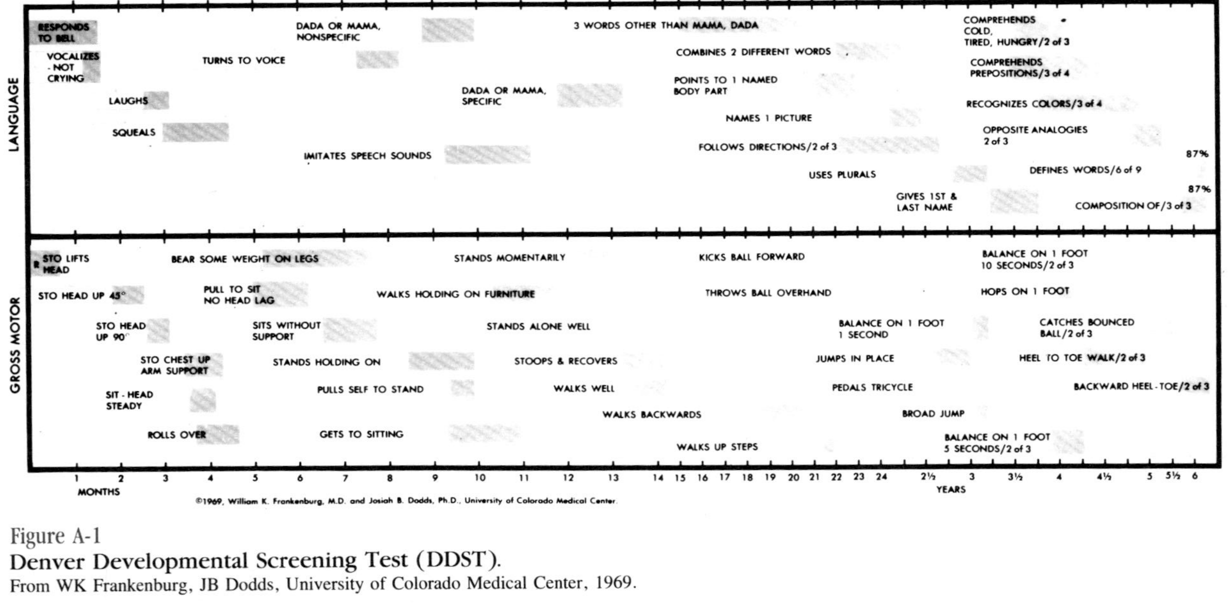

Figure A-1
Denver Developmental Screening Test (DDST).
From WK Frankenburg, JB Dodds, University of Colorado Medical Center, 1969.

DATE:
NAME:
DIRECTIONS BIRTH DATE:
HOSP. NO.:

1. Try to get child to smile by smiling, talking or waving to him. Do not touch him.
2. When child is playing with toy, pull it away from him. Pass if he resists.
3. Child does not have to be able to tie shoes or button in the back.
4. Move yarn slowly in an arc from one side to the other, about 6" above child's face. Pass if eyes follow 90° to midline. (Past midline; 180°)
5. Pass if child grasps rattle when it is touched to the backs or tips of fingers.
6. Pass if child continues to look where yarn disappeared or tries to see where it went. Yarn should be dropped quickly from sight from tester's hand without arm movement.
7. Pass if child picks up raisin with any part of thumb and a finger.
8. Pass if child picks up raisin with the ends of thumb and index finger using an over hand approach.

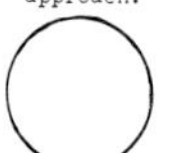
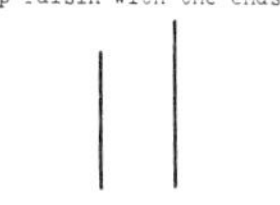
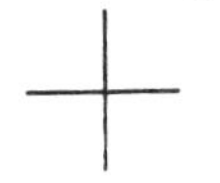

9. Pass any enclosed form. Fail continuous round motions.
10. Which line is longer? (Not bigger.) Turn paper upside down and repeat. (3/3 or 5/6)
11. Pass any crossing lines.
12. Have child copy first. If failed, demonstrate

When giving items 9, 11 and 12, do not name the forms. Do not demonstrate 9 and 11.

13. When scoring, each pair (2 arms, 2 legs, etc.) counts as one part.
14. Point to picture and have child name it. (No credit is given for sounds only.)

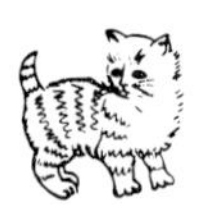
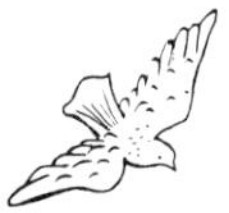
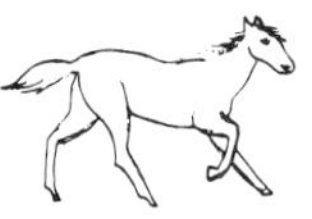
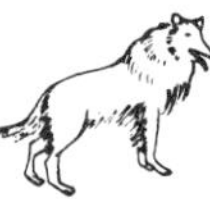
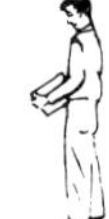

15. Tell child to: Give block to Mommie; put block on table; put block on floor. Pass 2 of 3. (Do not help child by pointing, moving head or eyes.)
16. Ask child: What do you do when you are cold? ..hungry? ..tired? Pass 2 of 3.
17. Tell child to: Put block <u>on</u> table; <u>under</u> table; <u>in front</u> of chair, <u>behind</u> chair. Pass 3 of 4. (Do not help child by pointing, moving head or eyes.)
18. Ask child: If fire is hot, ice is ?; Mother is a woman, Dad is a ?; a horse is big, a mouse is ?. Pass 2 of 3.
19. Ask child: What is a ball? ..lake? ..desk? ..house? ..banana? ..curtain? ..ceiling? ..hedge? ..pavement? Pass if defined in terms of use, shape, what it is made of or general category (such as banana is fruit, not just yellow). Pass 6 of 9.
20. Ask child: What is a spoon made of? ..a shoe made of? ..a door made of? (No other objects may be substituted.) Pass 3 of 3.
21. When placed on stomach, child lifts chest off table with support of forearms and/or hands.
22. When child is on back, grasp his hands and pull him to sitting. Pass if head does not hang back.
23. Child may use wall or rail only, not person. May not crawl.
24. Child must throw ball overhand 3 feet to within arm's reach of tester.
25. Child must perform standing broad jump over width of test sheet. (8-1/2 inches)
26. Tell child to walk forward, heel within 1 inch of toe. Tester may demonstrate. Child must walk 4 consecutive steps, 2 out of 3 trials.
27. Bounce ball to child who should stand 3 feet away from tester. Child must catch ball with hands, not arms, 2 out of 3 trials.
28. Tell child to walk backward, toe within 1 inch of heel. Tester may demonstrate. Child must walk 4 consecutive steps, 2 out of 3 trials.

<u>DATE AND BEHAVIORAL OBSERVATIONS</u> (how child feels at time of test, relation to tester, attention span, verbal behavior, self-confidence, etc,):

Figure A-2

Directions for numbered items on Denver Developmental Screening Test (DDST) and DDST-Revised.

From WK Frankenburg, JB Dobbs, University of Colorado Medical Center, 1969.

Appendix B
Growth Charts

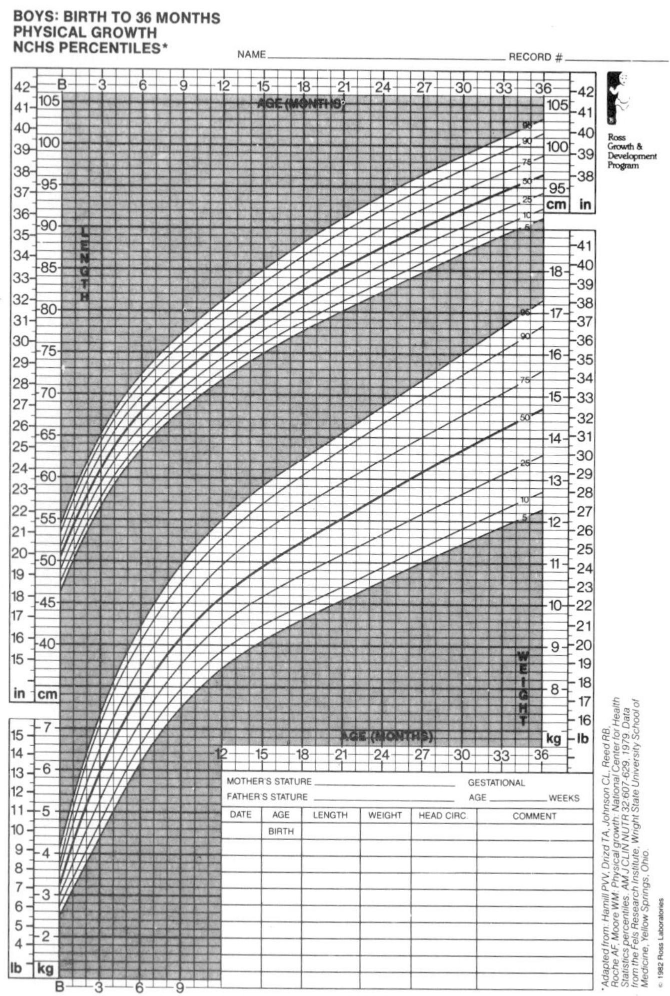

Figure B-1
Boys physical growth: birth to 36 months.

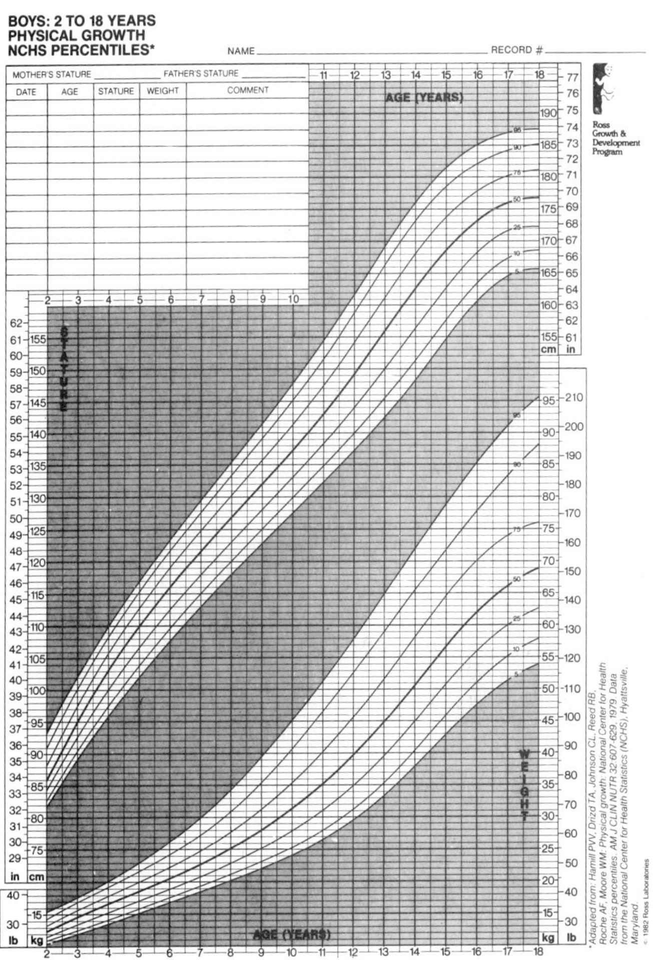

Figure B-2
Boys physical growth: 2 to 18 years.

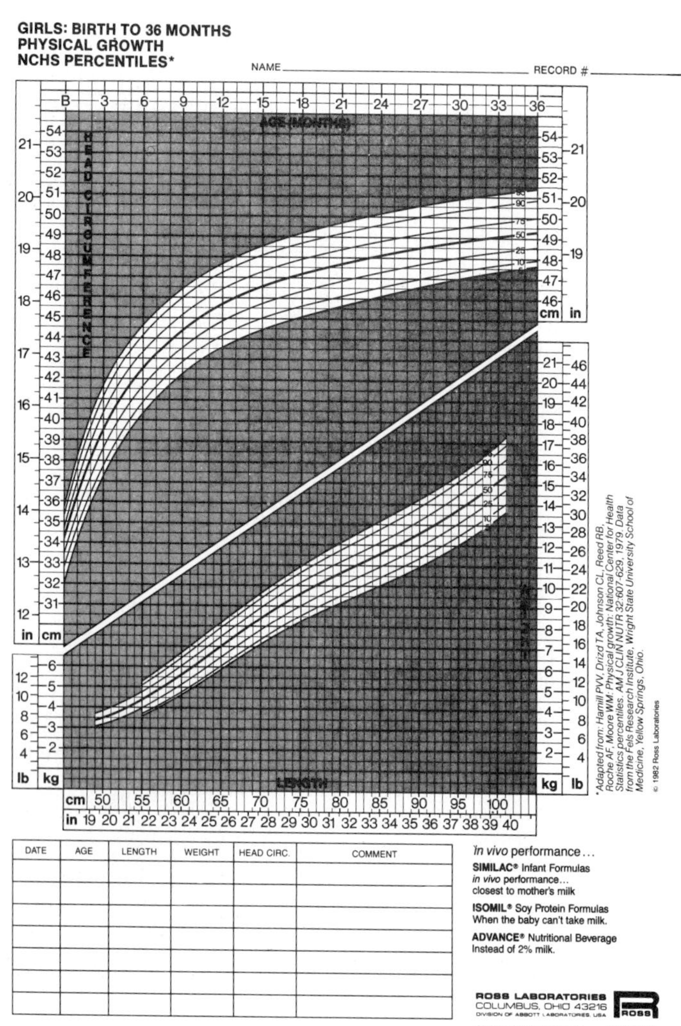

Figure B-3
Girls physical growth: birth to 36 months.

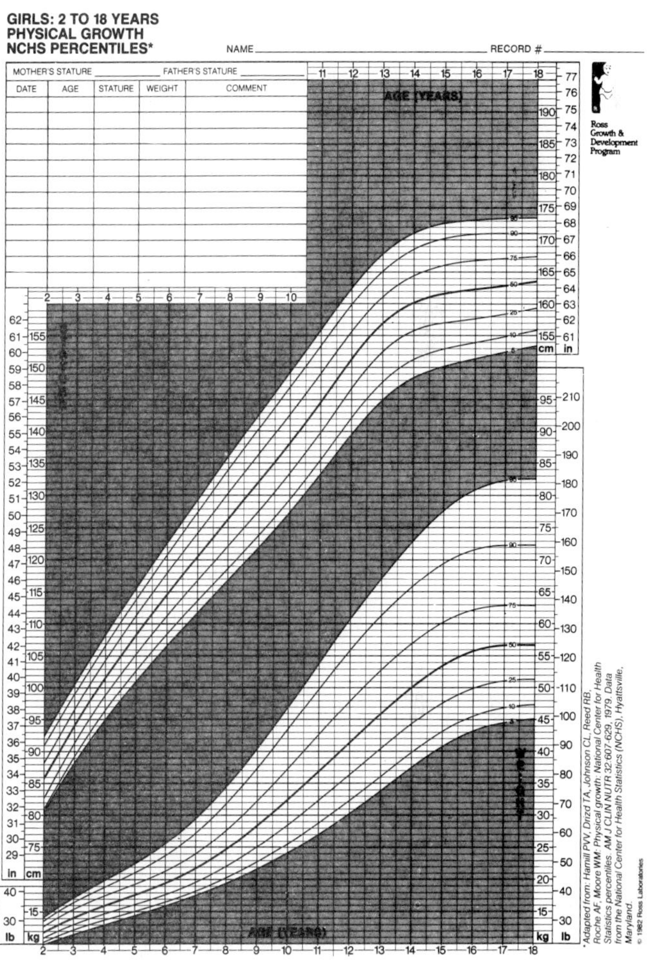

Figure B-4
Girls physical growth: 2-18 years.

Appendix C Normal Laboratory Values

Table C-1 Hematology

Test	Age/Sex	Reference Range	
		Conventional Values	International Units
		% Packed Cells	Volume Fraction
Hematocrit (Hct)	Infant:	28-48	0.28-0.48
	Child (6-12 yr)	33-47	0.33-0.47
	Adolescent: Male	37-54	0.37-0.54
	Female	36-47	0.36-0.47
		gm/dl	mmol/L
Hemoglobin (Hb)	Infant	9-14	1.40-2.17
	Child (6-12 yr)	11.5-15.5	1.78-2.40
	Adolescent: Male	13-16	2.02-2.48
	Female	12-16	1.86-2.48
		Million Cells/mm^3 (μL)	$\times 10^{12}$ Cells/L

Continued.

Table C-1 Hematology—cont'd

Test	Age/Sex	Reference Range	
		Conventional Values	International Units
Red blood cell count (erythrocyte count)	Infant	2.7-5.4	2.7-5.4
	Child (2-12 yr)	3.9-5.3	3.9-5.3
	Adolescent: Male	4.7-6.1	4.7-6.1
	Female	4.1-5.4	4.1-5.4
		$\times 10^3/mm^3$ (μL)	$\times 10^9/L$
Platelet count (thrombocyte count)	Newborn	84-478	84-478
	Thereafter	150-400	150-400
Blood indices		μm^3	fL
Mean corpuscular volume (MCV)	Infant	70-86	70-86
	Child (6-12 yr)	77-96	77-96
	Adolescent: Male (12-18 yr)	80-94	80-94
	Female (12-18 yr)	81-99	81-99
		pg/Cell	fmol/Cell
Mean corpuscular hemoglobin (MCH)	2-6 mo	25-35	0.39-0.54
	6-24 mo	23-31	0.36-0.48

	Thereafter	25-34	0.39-0.54
		%Hb/Cell	mmol
Mean corpuscular hemoglobin concentration (MCHC)	Infant	29-36	4.50-5.58
	Thereafter	31-37	4.81-5.74
		%	Number Fraction
Reticulocyte count	Infant	0.3-3.1	0.003-0.031
	Thereafter	0.5-2.5	0.005-0.025
		mm/hr	mm/hr
Sedimentation rate (erythrocyte sedimentation rate or ESR)	Child	3-13	3-13
	Thereafter: Male	1-15	1-15
	Female	1-20	1-20
		× 1000 Cells/mm^3 (μL)	× 10^9 Cells/L
White blood cell count (leukocyte count)	1 mo	5.0-19.5	5.0-19.5
	1-7 yr	5.5-17.5	5.5-17.5
	8-13 yr	4.5-13.5	4.5-13.5
	Thereafter	4.5-11.0	4.5-11.0
Differential white blood cell count		%	Number Fraction
Neutrophils (segmented and bands)	Infant	23	0.23
	Child	31-61	0.31-0.61
	Thereafter	54-75	0.54-0.75

Continued.

Table C-1 Hematology—cont'd

Test	Age/Sex	Reference Range	
		Conventional Values	International Units
Eosinophils		1-3	0.01-0.03
Basophils		0-0.75	0-0.0075
Lymphocytes	Infant	61	0.61
	Child	28-48	0.28-0.48
	Thereafter	25-40	0.25-0.40
Monocytes	Infant	5	0.05
	Child	4-4.5	0.04-0.045
	Thereafter	2-8	0.02-0.08
Bleeding time	Infant/child/adolescent	1-6 min	1-6 min

Clotting time	Infant/child/adolescent	5-8 min	5-8 min
Prothrombin time (PT), one stage, quick	Infant/child/adolescent	11-15 sec	11-15 sec
Partial thromboplastin time (PTT), nonactivated	Infant/child/adolescent	24-40 sec	24-40 sec
Partial thromboplastin time (APTT), activated	Infant (to 6 mo)	<90 sec	<90 sec
	Thereafter	25-35 sec	25-35 sec
Fibrinogen level	Infant/child/adolescent	mg/dl 200-450	2.00-4.50

Table C-2 Normal cerebrospinal fluid values

Test	Age/Sex	Reference Range	
		Conventional Values	International Units
		mmol/L	mmol/L
Chloride	Infant/child/adolescent	118-132	118-132
		mg/dL	mmol/L
Glucose	Infant/child/adolescent	40-70	2.2-3.9
Differential leukocyte count		%	Number Fraction
Lymphocytes		62 ± 34	0.62 ± 0.34
Monocytes		36 ± 20	0.36 ± 0.20
Neutrophils		2 ± 5	0.02 ± 0.05
Eosinophils		Rare	Rare
		mg/dL	mg/L
Protein, total		8-32	80-320
		mmol/L	mmol/L
Sodium		118-132	118-132
Specific gravity		1.007-1.009	1.007-1.009

Table C-3 Blood chemistry values

Test	Specimen	Age/Sex	Reference Range	
			Conventional Values	International Units
Acetone			mg/dL	mmol/L
Semiquantative	Serum/plasma		Negative	Negative
Quantitative			0.3-2.0	0.05-0.34
			U/L	U/L
Alkaline phosphatase (SKI method)	Serum	Infant	50-155	50-155
		Child	20-150	20-150
		Adolescent	20-70	20-70
			U/L	U/L
Amylase	Serum	Infant	5-65	5-65
		Thereafter (>1 yr)	25-125	25-125
	Urine (timed specimen)		1-17 U/hr	1-17 U/hr
Bilirubin			mg/dL	μmol/L
Total	Serum	Infant/child/adolescent	0.2-1.0	3.4-17.1
Direct (conjugated)	Serum	Infant/child/adolescent	0.0-0.2	0-3.4
			mg/dL	mmol/L

Continued.

Table C-3 Blood chemistry values—cont'd

Test	Specimen	Age/Sex	Reference Range	
			Conventional Values	International Units
Calcium	Serum, plasma	Infant/child/adolescent	4.48-4.92	1.12-2.70
Ionized	whole blood			
Total	Serum	Child	8.8-10.8	2.2-2.70
		Thereafter	8.4-10.2	2.1-2.55
			µg/dL	µmol/L
β-carotene	Serum	Infant	20-70	0.37-1.30
		Child	40-130	0.74-2.42
		Thereafter	60-200	1.12-3.72
			mmol/L	mmol/L
Chloride	Serum/plasma	Infant/child/adolescent	90-106	90-106
	Urine	Infant	2-10	2-10
		Child	15-40	15-40
		Adolescent	110-250	110-250
	Sweat	Normal	0-35	0-35
		Marginal	35-70	35-70
		Cystic fibrosis	70-200	70-200
			mg/dL	mmol/L

Cholesterol, total	Serum	Infant	70-175	1.81-4.53
		Child	120-200	3.11-5.18
		Adolescent	120-210	3.11-5.44
			μg/dL	μmol/L
Copper	Serum	Infant/child	30-190	4.7-29.83
		Adolescent	70-155	10.99-24.34
			μg/dL	nmol/L
Cortisol	Plasma, serum	Infant/child	5-23	138-635
		Adolescent	2-15	55-413
			U/L	U/L
Creatine kinase (CK, CPK)	Serum	Infant/child/adolescent: Male	12-70	12-70
		Female	10-50	10-50
		(higher in blacks and after exercise)		
			mg/dL	μmol/L
Creatinine	Serum, plasma	Infant	0.2-0.4	18-35
		Child	0.3-0.7	27-62
		Adolescent	0.5-1.0	44-88
			mg/dL	mmol/L
Fatty acids, free	Serum, plasma	Children/obese adults	<31	<1.10
			g/day	g/day
Fecal fat	Feces	0-6 yr	<2	<2

Table C-3 Blood chemistry values—cont'd

Test	Specimen	Age/Sex		Reference Range		
				Conventional Values	International Units	
		Thereafter		<7	<7	
				ng/ml	θg/L	
Ferritin	Serum	1 mo		200-600	200-600	
		2-5 mo		50-200	50-200	
		6 mo-15 yr		7-140	7-140	
				ng/ml	nmol/L	
Folate	Serum	Infant/child/adolescent		1.8-9	4.1-20.4	
				mg/dL	mmol/L	
Galactose	Serum	Infant/child/adolescent		<5	<0.28	
				mg/dL	mmol/L	
Glucose	Serum	Child		60-100	3.3-5.5	
		Adolescent		70-105	3.9-5.8	
	Urine (qualitative)			Negative	Negative	
			mg/dL	mg/dL	mmol/L	mmol/L
		Time (min)	Normal	Diabetic	Normal	Diabetic
Glucose tolerance (GTT)		Fasting	70-105	>115	3.9-5.8	>6.4
Dosage		60	120-160	>200	6.7-8.8	≥11
0-18 mo 2.5 gm/kg		90	100-140	>200	5.6-7.8	≥11

18 mo-3 yr	2.0 gm/kg	120	65-120	>140	3.6-6.7	≥7.8
3-12 yr	1.75 gm/kg					
>12 yr	1.25 gm/kg (maximum 100 gm)					
				mg/day	μmol/day	
17-Hydroxycorticosteroids (17-OHCS)	Urine 24 hr	Infant		0.5-1.0	1.4-2.8	
		Child		1.0-5.6	2.8-15.5	
		Adolescent: Male		3.0-10.0	8.2-27.6	
		Female		2.0-8.0	5.5-22	
				mg/dL	mg/L	
Immunoglobulin A (IgA)	Serum	1-6 mo		3-82	30-820	
		6 mo-2 yr		14-108	140-1080	
		2-6 yr		23-190	230-1900	
		6-12 yr		29-270	290-2700	
		12-16 yr		81-232	810-2320	
				mg/dL	μmol/L	
Immunoglobulin D (IgD)	Serum	Child/adolescent		0-8	0-0.44	
				IU/mL	kIU/L	
Immunoglobulin E (IgE)	Serum	Male		0-230	0-230	
		Female		0-170	0-170	
				mg/dL	g/L	
Imunoglobulin G (IgG)	Serum	1-6 mo		300-1000	3-10	
		6 mo-2 yr		500-1200	5-12	
		2-6 yr		500-1300	5-13	

Continued.

Table C-3 Blood chemistry values—cont'd

Test	Specimen	Age/Sex	Reference Range	
			Conventional Values	International Units
		6-12 yr	700-1650	7-16.5
		12-16 yr	700-1550	7-15.5
			µg/dL	µmol/L
Iron	Serum	Infant	40-100	7.16-17.90
		Child	50-120	8.95-21.48
		Adolescent: Male	50-160	8.95-28.64
		Female	40-150	7.16-26.85
		Intoxicated child	280-2550	50.12-456.5
		Fatally poisoned child	>1800	322.2
			µg/dL	µmol/IL
Iron binding capacity	Serum	Infant	100-400	17.90-71.60
		Thereafter	250-400	44.75-71.60
			µg/dL	µmol/L
Lead	Whole blood	Child	<30	<1.45
		Adolescent	<40	<1.93
		Toxic	≥100	≥2.90
			U/mL	U/L

Lipase (Tietz method)	Serum	Child/adolescent	0.1-1.0	28-280
			mEq/L	mmol/L
Magnesium	Serum	Infant/child/adolescent	1.3-2.1	0.65 ± 1.05
			mOsm/kg H_2O	
Osmolality	Serum		275-295	
			mg/dL	mmol/L
Phenylalanine	Serum	Infant/child/adolescent	0.8-1.8	0.05-0.11
			mg/dL	mmol/L
Phosphorus, inorganic	Serum	Infant/child	4.5-6.5	1.45-2.1
		Adolescent	3.0-4.5	0.97-1.45
			mmol/L	mmol/L
Potassium	Serum	Infant	4.1-5.3	4.1-5.3
		Child	3.4-4.7	3.4-4.7
		Adolescent	3.5-5.3	3.5-5.3
			g/dL	g/L
Protein, total	Serum	Child	6.2-8.0	62.0-80.0
		Adolescent	6.0-8.0	60.0-80.0
			mg/dL	mmol/L
Salicylates	Serum, plasma	Therapeutic	15-30	1.1-2.2
		Toxic	>30	>2.2

Continued.

Table C-3 Blood chemistry values—cont'd

Test	Specimen	Age/Sex	Reference Range	
			Conventional Values	International Units
			mmol/L	mmol/L
Sodium	Serum	Infant	139-146	139-146
		Child	138-145	138-145
		Adolescent	135-148	135-148
			μg/dL	nmol/L
Thiamine (vitamin B_1)	Whole blood		0-2.0	0.75-4
			μU/L	μU/L
Thyroid-stimulating hormone (hTSH)	Serum, plasma	Infant/child/adolescent	2-11	2-11
			mg/dL	g/L
Transferrin	Serum	Infant/child/adolescent	200-400	2.0-4.0
			mg/dL	g/L
Triglycerides (TG: neutral fat)	Serum	Infant	5-40	0.05-0.40
		Adolescent	30-150	0.30-1.50

		Male	40-160	0.40-1.60
		Female	35-135	0.35-1.35
			mg/dL	mmol/L
Tyrosine	Serum	Infant/child/adolescent	0.8-1.3	0.044-0.07
			mg/dL	mmolurea/L
Urea nitrogen	Serum, plasma	Infant/child	5-18	1.8-6.4
		Adolescent	7-18	2.5-6.4
			mg/dl	µmol/L
Uric acid	Serum	Child	2.0-5.5	119-327
		Adolescent: Male	3.5-7.2	208-438
		Female	3.0-8.2	178-488
			µm/dL	µmol/L
Vitamin A	Serum	Child	30-80	1.22-2.62
		Adolescent	30-65	1.05-2.27
			pg/ml	pmol/L
Vitamin B_{12}	Serum	Infant/child/adolescent	140-900	103-454
			mg/dL	µmol/L
Vitamin C	Serum	Infant/child/adolescent	0.6-2.0	34-113
			µg/mL	µmol/L
Vitamin E	Serum	Infant/child	5-20	17.6-46.4

Table C-4 Blood gas determinations

Determination	Age	Reference Range	
		Conventional Values	International Units
pH	Child	7.33-7.43	7.33-7.43
	Adolescent	7.35-7.45	7.35-7.45
		mm Hg	k/Pa
Pco_2	Child/adolescent	35-45	4.7-6.0
Pao_2	Child/adolescent	75-100	10.0-13.3
		mmol/L	mmol/L
Hco_3, venous	Infant/child/adolescent (arterial approximately 2 mmol/L lower)	22-29	22-29
		mmol/L	mmol/L
Base excess	Infant	(−7)-(−1)	(−7)-(−1)
	Child	(−4)-(+2)	(−4)-(+2)
	Thereafter	(−3)-(+3)	(−3)-(+3)

Table C-5 Urinalysis

Test	Age/Sex	Reference Range	
		Conventional Values	International Units
Bilirubin		Negative	Negative
		Clean Catch	Catheterization
Colony count	Infant/child	<1000	100
	Thereafter	<10,000	100
Glucose, qualitative		Negative	Negative
Microscopy		Per High-Power Field	
Leukocytes		0-4	
Erythrocytes		Rare	
Casts		Rare	
Occult blood		Negative	Negative
Osmolality		mOsm/kg H_2O	
Random	Infant/child/adolescent	50-1400	
24-Hour	Infant/child/adolescent	300-900	
		µmol/L	µmol/L
pH	Infant/child/adolescent	4.5-8	0.01-32.0

Appendix D
Immunization Schedules for Infants and Children

Table D-1 Recommended immunization schedule for infants*

Age	Immunizations	Comments
2 mo	DPT	Diphtheria-pertussis-tetanus (vaccine). Combined vaccine given to children younger than 7 years of age. May produce localized redness, swelling, and tenderness at injection site. Fever common in first 12-24 hours. Encephalitis from pertussis is rare.
	OPV (Sabin vaccine)	Trivalent oral live polio vaccine. Vaccine-induced paralytic disease is a possible but rare complication. Inactivated poliovirus vaccine (IPV) given by injection to infants and children with immune deficiency disorders.
	Hib	Haemophilus influenzae b conjugate (vaccine). Dosage schedule depends on whether HbOC or PRP-OMP is used and on age of child. Localized swelling and redness at injection site are common.

*Schedule may vary slightly depending on locale.

**Infants and children infected with HIV should receive DPT, inactivated oral polio vaccine (in place of oral polio vaccine), Hib, and pneumococcal vaccines. Household contacts should also receive the inactivated polio vaccine. Because of the high incidence of measles in children with HIV infection, MMR should be given.

Continued.

Table D-1 Recommended immunization schedule for infants —cont'd

Age	Immunizations	Comments
4 mo	DPT, OPV, Hib	
6 mo	DPT	
	OPV (optional)	
	Hib (if using HbOC series)	
12 mo	Hib (if using PRP-OMP series)	
15 mo	MMR	Live attenuated measles-mumps rubella (vaccine); may give simultaneously with DPT and OPV at 15 months. MMR may produce fever, rash 10-14 days following administration.
	Hib (if using HbOC)	
18 mo	DPT, OPV	
4-6 yr	DPT, OPV	
14-16	Td	Tetanus-diphtheria (toxoid) with lower diphtheria dose than in DPT or DT. Repeat every 10 years.
	OPV	

Table D-2 Recommended immunization schedule for infants and children not immunized in first year of life

Age	Immunization	Comments
59 Months or Younger		
First visit	DPT, OPV, MMR*	MMR if child is 15 months age.
Interval after first visit		
1 mo	Hib	HBOC or PRP-OMP may be given if the child is 13-59 months; PRP-D is approved for use in infants 15 months or older.
2 mo	DPT, OPV	
4 mo	DPT, OPV (optional)	
10-16 mo	DPT, OPV	OPV not necessary if third dose given earlier.
4-6 yr	DPT, OPV	DPT and OPV not necessary if fourth doses given after age 4 years.
14-16 yr	Td	Repeat every 10 years.
5 Years or Older		
First visit	Td, OPV, MMR	
Interval after first visit		
2 mo	Td, OPV	
18-14 mo	Td, OPV	
14-16 yr	Td	Repeat every 10 years.

*Definitions as in Table D-1.

Appendix E Sample Documentation of a Child Health History

Name: Sarah R. Age: 32 months Sex: female

Address: 214 Fifth Avenue Telephone: 567-9931 (parent's home)

Date of Admission: December 1 Telephone: 572-9771 (father's workplace)

Medical Diagnosis: bilateral otitis media (BOM) Allergies: None known

Source of History: mother (Michelle) and father (Jason)

Chief Complaints

"Pale for about 3 days. . . .not eating. . . .runny nose for a week. . . .cranky." Doctor says Sarah may have an "earache." Child crying on admission and saying "owie, owie."

Present Illness

Child has been sick for about 1 week. "Ran temperature for 2 days" and "had cough and runny nose. . . .Just didn't come around. . . .didn't eat." Mother says she is really tired because she has been up with Sarah for about 3 nights. Worried about impact of BOM on Sarah's hearing; had niece who had a ruptured "eardrum" and had "speech problems." Dad feels mother may be "babying" Sarah because she spends so much time with Sarah.

Past Health History

Birth history:

Patient delivered by normal, uncomplicated, vaginal delivery. Mom and Sarah in hospital for 2 days following delivery. No obvious congenital abnormalities detected at birth.

Feeding history:

Child "slow to gain" as an infant. Weight at birth 3.4 kg. Weight at one year 7.8 kg. "Picky eater" and "had to have formula changed a lot" because of "gas and crying." Cereal introduced at 4 months, fruits at 6 months, vegetables at 7 months, and full diet with homogenized milk by 9 months, with no adverse effects. Now eats nearly everything except peas. Eats "a lot." Takes a chewable multivitamin daily. Weaned from bottle at 18 months.

Dietary recall:

In the last 24 hours, child has had "about" 4 oz of milk, 8 oz of juice, bowl of soup, 2 crackers, an ice cream cone, and "2 spoonsful" of rice.

Elimination history:

"Constipated a lot when on formula . . . poops were hard and smelly . . . "Since going on homogenized milk has been better . . . still has hard stools if she drinks too much milk." Mom "limits" milk intake to about 16 oz a day and encourages child to drink juice. Child prefers juice to fruit or vegetables.

Childhood illnesses:

Chickenpox at 1 year. Surgery for pyloric stenosis at 10 days.

Immunizations:

2 mo—DPT, OPV
4 mo—DPT, OPV
6 mo—DPT No untoward reactions
15 mo—MMR
18 mo—DPT, OPV, Hib

Current medications:

Tylenol 80 mg (liquid) at 2 PM (2 hours ago) for fever.

Growth and Development History

General development:

No delays noted on Denver II.

Physical growth:

Weight pattern noted above. All "baby teeth" in by 21 months. Current weight 14.8 kg; height 51 cm. Completely toilet trained. Goes to bathroom on own; will ask to go "#1" or "#2."

Gross motor development:

Rolled over from back to front and front to back by 5 months. Walked at 11 months. Able to jump with both feet and to stand on one foot momentarily.

Fine motor development:

Holds crayon with fingers; able to copy circle; enjoys coloring.

Sleep:

Child established uninterrupted nighttime sleep pattern at 6 months, but reverted to frequent night awakenings at 8 months. Mom says no changes in family or environment at this time. Since 8 months sleeps about 10 hours a night with frequent awakenings which have no pattern. Child sometimes confused and crying when she awakens but at other times is calm. Mother responds to awakenings by taking child to bathroom and giving her a drink. If child does not immediately settle to crib after this, mom takes her into the family bed. Child does not have afternoon naps; goes down for night between 9 and 10 PM and gets up for day around 7:30 AM; generally is held and read to before bedtime; takes pink baby blanket to bed.

Language development:

First word at 9 months. First phrases after 24 months. Vocalization on admission limited primarily to "owie" and crying; however, mom states that child is usually very talkative, easy to understand. Has trouble with "l's" and "y's"; for example, says "lellow" for yellow. Uses sentences of 4 or 5 words. "Gets upset if you don't understand her and sulks."

Social development:

Recognizes familiar people, objects, and places. Initially shy with adults. Aggressive with other children; "bites and hits when she wants something." Parents use "time out" if child is aggressive or misbehaving. Dad feels spanking would be more effective; mom disagrees. Able to feed and dress self almost completely. "Very independent." "Occasional temper tantrums: screams and throws herself to ground. . .usually when meals are late." Has developed fear of "monsters."

Cognitive development:

Alert; follows instructions to "sit up here" or "lay down."

Personal/Social History

Family has well-defined parameters. Parents see themselves as "separate" from their families and able to set own patterns of discipline. Michelle sees her mother's depression as sometimes troublesome and says her mother demands Michelle's time but has little time for her granddaughter. Jason and Michelle express conflict over discipline of Sarah. Both state that they have difficulty solving problems such as discipline because Jason gets "mad and walks out" and then Michelle withdraws for "awhile," which makes Jason mad. Family communication is "open" around matters involving household tasks and responsibilities but there is more difficulty with expressing emotion. Discipline of Sarah largely involves "time out." Father feels Sarah rules her mother sometimes, a perception not shared by Michelle. Couple states they have a wide network of friends, including Sarah's babysitter, to whom Sarah is "very attached." Michelle is a sales rep for a medical supply company; some college education. Jason is an engineer and has a university degree. See genogram and ecomap (Figure E-1) for further information regarding internal and external family structures.

Systems Review

1. General:
   Palc, tired-looking child; alert; clings to mother when first approached; moves without difficulty.
   Temperature: 38.2 (A)
   Pulse: 130 (apical)/min; regular
   Respiration: 30/min
   Blood pressure: 98/64
   Weight: 14.8 (clothed)
   Height: 51 cm (no shoes)

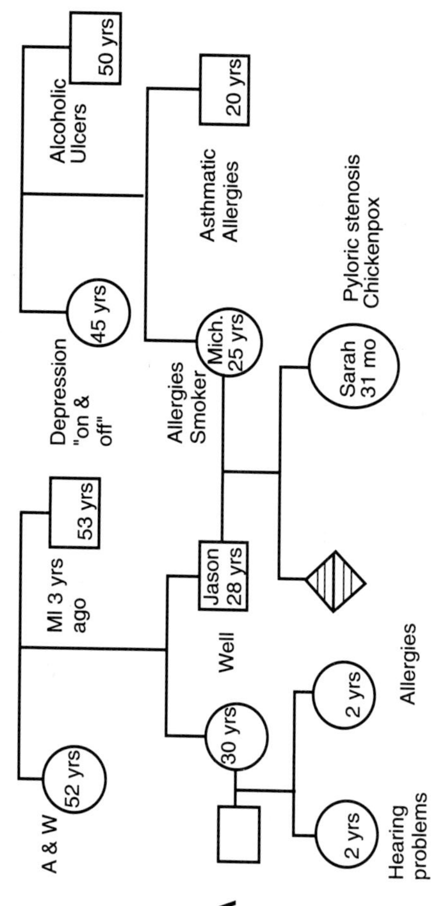
A
A & W
52 yrs
MI 3 yrs ago
53 yrs
Depression "on & off"
45 yrs
Alcoholic Ulcers
50 yrs
30 yrs
Well
Jason 28 yrs
Allergies Smoker
Mich. 25 yrs
Asthmatic Allergies
20 yrs
2 yrs
Hearing problems
2 yrs
Allergies
Sarah 31 mo
Pyloric stenosis Chickenpox

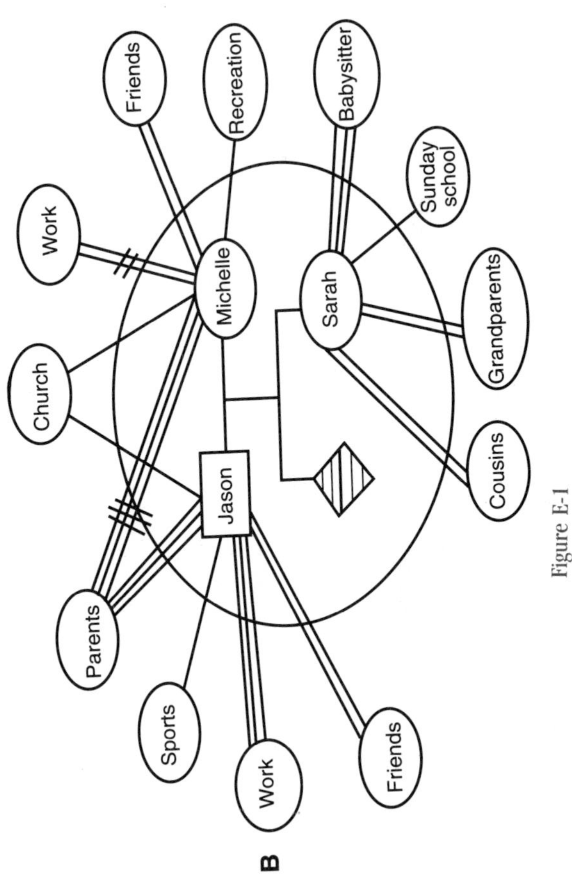

Figure E-1
A, Genogram and **B**, ecomap.

Systems Review

2. Integumen:
   Skin: Pale, warm; slightly dry in arm creases; elastic; no edema. Lesion approximately 2.5 cm in diameter, red, dry, and raised on left medial forearm "due to fall from tricycle 2 weeks ago." Indented area "old chickenpox scar" (approximately 2 mm) near left eyebrow.

   Mucous membranes: Reddened, moist.

   Nailbeds: Pink, texture firm, no clubbing; tooth imprints on left index finger "due to sucking."

   Hair/scalp: Hair clean, soft, abundant on scalp. Scalp clean, no lesions.

3. Head and neck:
   Head: Normocephalic.

   Neck: Full ROM, strong symmetrically; trachea at midline; thyroid not palpable. Firm, warm, diffuse nodes palpated in preauricular, submandibular, occipital, and cervical regions.

4. Ears:
   Auricle: No lesions, canals clean and free of cerumen.

   Otoscopic examination: Drums bilaterally intact, red, and bulging; landmarks not present.

   Hearing: Child asked for directions to be repeated on nearly every occasion. Rinne and Weber's Tests: unable to gain child's cooperation sufficiently to gain accurate assessments.

5. Eyes:
   Vision: Able to name 4 of 7 cards on two tries at 4.6 m.

   Extraocular movement: No deviation with cover test, light reflex equal. Unable to gain cooperation in fields of vision testing.

   Conjunctivia: Clear.

Systems Review

Sclerae: Clear, white.

Iris: Blue, round.

Pupils: PERRLA.

Ophthalmoscopic examination: Disc round, creamy white; macular areas normal; normal veins and arteries.

Lacrimal system: No swelling, excess tearing.

Corneal reflex: Present.

6. Face, nose, and oral cavity:
Face, nose, and facial movements: Symmetrical; child solemn but smiles with encouragement; marked shadows under both eyes; external nares excoriated, green thick nasal discharge present; no pain on palpation of cheeks and areas above eyebrows; septum slightly deviated to left.

Oral cavity: Lips dry, pale, and slightly cracked; oral membranes moist, pink, no lesions.
Gums: No edema or swelling.
Teeth: Clean, all present. Both upper, central incisors protrude slightly.
Tonsils red and almost to uvula; adenoids visible; voice hoarse.

7. Thorax and lungs:

Thorax slightly oval, symmetrical at rest. No indrawings. Respirations diaphragmatic. Tactile fremitus equal bilaterally. Vesicular sounds heard through lung fields. No adventitious sounds.

8. Cardiovascular system:
Heart: PMI in 4 ICS; no abnormal pulsations palpated, $S_1 > S_2$ in mitral, tricuspid areas and at Erb's point. Systolic murmer heard in 3rd ICS.

Vascular system: Radial and peripheral pulses equal, regular, and strong.

Systems Review

9. Abdomen:

Healed scar in epigastric region (pyloric stenosis), abdomen protruberant, symmetrical; no bulging, bowel sounds 4 to 5/min in each quadrant; firm mass palpated in LLQ (last bowel movement 4 days ago), no hernias.

10. Genitourinary/reproductive system:
Breasts: Nipples symmetrical, aerola pink; no discharge.

Genitalia: Labia approximate and are intact; vagina pink, no discharge.

11. Musculoskeletal system:

Muscular development and mass normal for age; movements symmetric; gait normal; feet slightly flattened; all digits present; joints nontender, not swollen; full range of motion; Kernig's sign negative.

12. Nervous system:
Mental status: Child follows directions appropriately when direction repeated.

Cranial nerve function: Not done.

Motor function: Muscle strength equal and symmetrical.

Related Nursing Diagnoses

Anxiety: Related to hospitalization; pain.

Constipation: Related to decreased fluid and food intake; decreased mobility; and food preferences.

Communication, impaired verbal: Related to fear; anxiety; and decreased hearing abilities.

Family processes, alterations in: Related to child with infection; conflict between parents related to childrearing practices.

Fear: Related to hospitalization; fantasies.

Fluid volume deficit, potential: Related to reduced oral intake.

Knowledge deficit: Related to establishment of sleep patterns in toddlers; parenting practices.

Nutrition, altered: less than body requirements related to loss of appetite.

Pain related to pressure caused by inflammatory process and discomfort in swallowing.

Parental role conflict: Related to dysfunctional communication and problem solving around discipline issues.

Sleep pattern disturbance: Related to fears; trained night crying; and/or pain.

Appendix F Bibliography

Adams FN, Landau EM: What are healthy blood pressures for children? *Pediatrics* 681:268-270, 1981.

Adler J: Patient assessment: abnormalities of the heartbeat, *Am J Nurs* 77:647-673, 1977.

American Academy of Pediatrics: Report of the committee on infectious diseases, Elk Grove, Ill, 1991, The Academy.

Aynsley-Green A, Pickering D: Use of central and peripheral temperature measurements in care of the critically ill child, *Arch Dis Child* 49:477-481, 1973.

Baker NC et al: The effect of thermometer and length of time inserted on oral temperature measurements of afebrile subjects, *Nurs Res* 33:(2):109-111, 1984.

Barber N, Kilmon CA: Reactions to tympanic temperature measurement in an ambulatory care setting, *Ped Nurs* 15:477-481, 1989.

Barness LA: *Manual of pediatric physical diagnosis,* Chicago, 1980, Mosby–Year Book.

Bates B: *A guide to physical examination,* Philadelphia, 1983, JB Lippincott.

Beck CM et al: *Mental health-psychiatric nursing,* ed 3, St Louis, 1988, Mosby–Year Book.

Beecroft PC, Redick S: Possible complications of intramuscular injections on the pediatric unit, *Ped Nurs* 15:333-336, 1989.

Bellack JP, Bamford PA: *Nursing assessment and health promotion throughout the life span,* Englewood Cliffs, NJ, 1985, Prentice-Hall.

Berkey K, Hanson SM: Pocket guide to family assessment and intervention, St Louis, 1991, Mosby–Year Book.

Bliss-Holtz J: Comparison of rectal, axillary, and inguinal temperatures in full-term newborn infants, *WJNR* 38:85-87, 1989.

Boszormenyi-Nagy I, Spark G: *Invisible loyalties,* New York, 1984, Brunner/Mazel.

Bresnahan K et al: Prenatal cocaine use: impact on infants and mothers, *Ped Nurs* 17:123-129, 1991.

Broome ME: Preparation of children for painful procedures, *Ped Nurs* 16:490-496, 1990.

Brown MS: Vision tests for preschoolers, *Nursing '75* 5(5):72-75, 1975.

Brunner LS, Suddarth DS: *Lippincott manual of nursing practice,* Philadelphia, 1991, JB Lippincott.

Caufield C: A developmental approach to hearing screening in children, *Ped Nurs* 4:39-42, 1978.

Clark, MC: In what ways, if any, are child abusers different from other parents? *Health Visit* 62:268-270, 1989.

Clubb R: Chronic sorrow: adaptation patterns of parents with chronically ill children, *Ped Nurs* 17:461-465, 1991.

Cohen S: Patient assessment: examination of the male genitalia, *Am J Nurs* 79:689-712, 1979.

Cormier LS et al: Interviewing helping skills for health professionals, Monterey, Calif, 1984, Wadsworth Health Sciences Division.

Davies S et al: A comparison of mercury and digital thermometers, *J Adv Nurs* 11:535-543, 1986.

DeAngelis C: *Pediatric primary care,* ed 3, Boston, 1984, Little, Brown.

Derkes Y: Rashes: recognition and managmeent, *Nursing '78,* 8:54-59, 1978.

Dessertine PS: Those neglected heart sounds, *Ped Nurs* 3:18-20, 1977.

Doegnes M, Moorhouse M: *Nurses pocket guide: nursing diagnoses with interventions,* ed 2, Philadelphia, 1988, FA Davis.

Downs MP, Sliver NK: The "A.B.C.D." to H.E.A.R.: early identification in nursery, office, and office of the infant who is deaf, *Clin Pediatr* 11:563-565, 1972.

Dunst C et al: *Enabling and empowering families,* Cambridge, MA, 1988, Brookline Books.

Eddsteen S: Nutritional assessment in cancer cachexia, *Ped Nurs* 17:237-240, 1991.

Eggertsen SC et al: An updated protocol for pediatric health screening, *J Fam Pract* 10(1):25-37, 1980.

Engle MA: Heart sounds and murmurs in the diagnosis of heart disease, *Pediatr Ann* 10:18-31, March, 1987.

Erickson R: Oral temperature differences in relation to thermometer and technique, *Nurs Res* 29:157-160, 1980.

Faux SA et al: Intensive interviewing with children and adolescents, *WJNR* 10:180-194, 1988.

Frankenberg WK et al: The reliability and stability of the Denver Developmental Screening Test, *Child Dev* 42:1315, 1971.

Frankenberg WK et al: The revised Denver Developmental Screening Test: its accuracy as a screening instrument, *J Pediatr* 76:988-995, 1971.

Frankenberg WK et al: The Denver II: a major revison and restandardization of the Denver Developmental Screening tool, *Pediatrics* 89:91-97, 1992.

Fuller J, Schaller-Ayers J: *Health assessment: a nursing approach,* Philadelphia, 1990, JB Lippincott.

Gage RB: Consequences of children's exposure to spouse abuse, *Ped Nurs* 16:258-260, 1990.

Gordon M: *Manual of nursing diagnosis,* New York, 1982, McGraw-Hill.

Gryskiewicz JM, Huseby TC: The pediatric abdominal assessment: a multiple challenge, *Postgrad Med* 67:126-128, 1980.

Houck GM, King MC: Child maltreatment: family charactristics and developmental consequences, *Issues in Mental Health Nurs* 10:193-208, 1989.

Heiney SP: Helping children through painful procedures, *AJN* 91(11):20-24, 1991.

Hoeckelman RA et al: *Primary pediatric care,* St Louis, 1987, Mosby–Year Book.

Hole JW: *Human anatomy and physiology,* ed 2, Dubuque, 1981, William C Brown.

Hunter LP: Measurement of axillary temperatures in neonates. *WJNR* 13:324-335, 1991.

Johnson BH: Children's drawings as a projective technique, *Ped Nurs* 16:11-17, 1990.

Kahn-D'Angelo L: Serious head injury during the first year of life, *Phys Occup Ther Pediatr* 9(4):49-59, 1989.

Kaslow FW: *Voices in family psychiatry,* Newbury Park, Calif, 1990, Sage.

Kelley SJ et al: Birth outcomes, health problems and neglect with prenatal exposure to cocaine, *Ped Nurs* 17:130-136, 1991.

Kim MJ et al: Pocket guide to nursing diagnoses, ed 4, St Louis, 1991, Mosby–Year Book.

Kluger M: Fever, *Pediatrics* 66:720-723, 1980.

Kresch MJ: Axillary temperature as a screening test for fever in children, *J Pediatr* 104:596-599, 1984.

Krowchuck H: Child abuser stereotypes: consensus among clinicians, *Appl Nurs Res* 2:35-39, 1989.

Leahey M, Wright LM: *Families and life-threatening illness,* Springhouse, PA, 1987, Springhouse.

Lefrancois GR: *Of children,* Belfmont, Calif, 1977, Wadsworth Publishing.

Levin BE, Lavi S: Perils of childhood immunization against measles, mumps, and rubella, *Ped Nurs* 17:159-161, 1991.

Lewin L: Establishing a therapeutic relationship with an abused child, *Ped Nurs* 16:263-264, 1990.

Malasanos L et al: *Health assessment,* ed 4, St Louis, 1990, Mosby–Year Book.

Marino BL, Lipshitz M: Temperament in infants and toddlers with cardiac disease, *Ped Nurs* 17:445-448, 1991.

Mechner F: Patient assessment: neurological examination, part 111, *Am J Nurs* 76:608-633, 1976.

Meeropol E: Parental needs assessment: a design for nurse specialist practice, *Ped Nurs* 17:456-458, 1991.

Mosby's medical and nursing dictionary, ed 2, St Louis, 1990, Mosby–Year Book.

Mott SR et al: *Nursing care of children and families: a holistic approach,* Menlo Park, Calif, 1985, Addison-Wesley.

Pagana K, Pagana TJ: *Diagnostic testing and nursing implications,* ed 3, St Louis, 1990, Mosby–Year Book.

Patrick ML et al: *Medical-surgical nursing,* Philadelphia, 1991, JB Lippincott.

Performing palpation, *Nursing '83* 13(1):68-69, 1983.

Performing percussion, *Nursing '83* 13(2):63-64, 1983.

Perry AG, Potter PA: *Clinical nursing skills and techniques,* ed 2, St Louis, 1990, Mosby–Year Book.

Pilleteri A: *Child health nursing: care of the growing family,* Boston, 1987, Little, Brown.

Pillsbury D: *Manual of dermatology,* Philadelphia, 1971, WB Saunders.

Potter PA: *Pocket nurse guide to physical assessment,* ed 2, St Louis, 1990, Mosby–Year Book.

Quick G, Sicilio M: When should you suspect child abuse? A photographic guide: part 1: cutaneous lesions, *Consultant* 29(7):31-39, 1989.

Quick G, Sicilio M: When should you suspect child abuse? A photographic guide: part 3: neurologic manifestations, *Consultant* 29(7):70-76, 1989.

Recommendations for vaccine use, *MMWR* 40(RR-1):4-6, 1991.

Rogers J et al: Evaluation of use of tympanic membrane thermometer in pediatric patients, *Ped Nurs* 17:376-378, 1991.

Schroeder B, McEroy-Shields K: Visual acuity, binocular vision, and ocular muscle balance in VLBW children, *Ped Nurs* 17:30-33, 1991.

Schuster C, Ashburn S: *The process of human development: a holistic life-span appraoch,* Boston, 1986, Little, Brown.

Schweigger J et al: Oral assessment: how to do it, *Am J Nurs* 80:654-663, 1980.

Selikman J: The multiple focus of immune deficiency in children, *Ped Nurs* 16:351-355, 361, 1990.

Stanhope M, Lancaster J: *Community health nursing: process and practice for promoting health,* St Louis, 1992, Mosby–Year Book.

Stewart M et al: *Community health nursing in Canada,* Toronto, 1985, Gage Educational.

Stuart G, Sundeen SJ: *Principles and practice of psychiatric nursing,* St Louis, 1991, Mosby–Year Book.

Terkelson K: Toward a theory of family life cycle. In Carter EA, McGoldrick M, editors: *The family life cycle: a framework for family therapy,* New York, 1980, Gardner.

Tilkian SM, et al: *Clinical implications of laboratory tests,* ed 4, St Louis, 1987, Mosby–Year Book.

Waechter EN et al: *Nursing care of children,* ed 10, Philadelphia, 1985, JB Lippincott.

Wallace C, Farrington E: Pediatric drug information, *Ped Nurs* 17:372-374, 1991.

Wadsworth BJ: *Piaget's theory of cognitive and affective development,* ed 4, New York, 1989, Longman.

Walleck C: A neurological assessment procedure that won't make you nervous, *Nursing '82* 12(12):50-56, 1982.

Whaley LF, Wong DC: *Nursing care of infants and children,* St Louis, 1991, Mosby–Year Book.

Williams SR: *Nutrition and diet therapy,* St Louis, 1990, Mosby–Year Book.

Williams A: Nursing management of the child with AIDS, *Ped Nurs* 15:259-261, 1989.

Wilson CJ, Mason M: Preparation for routine physical examination, *Children's Health Care* 19:178-182, 1990.

Wong DC, Whaley LF: *Clinical manual of pediatric nursing,* St Louis, 1990, Mosby–Year Book.

Wright LM, Leahy M: *Nurses and families: a guide to family assessment and intervention,* Philadelphia, 1987, FA Davis.

Yoos L: A developmental approach to physical assessment, *Am J Maternal Child Nurs* 6:168-170, 1981.

Index

D

N